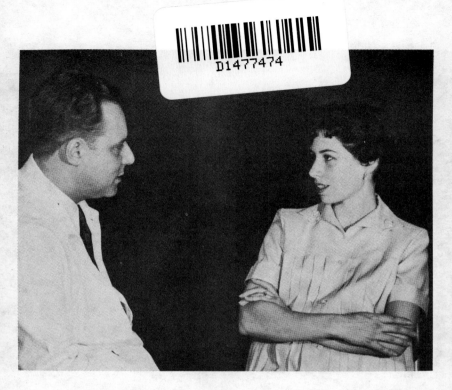

Your experience with hypnosis will begin sometime around the sixth month of your pregnancy, at which time your doctor will explain how hypnosis can help make the birth of your child a happier and healthier event.

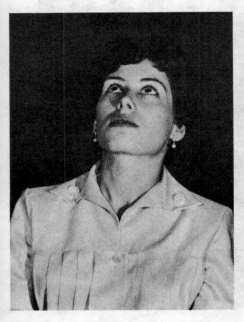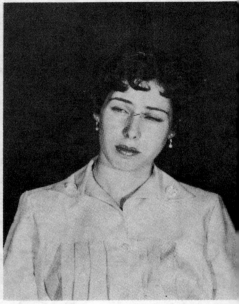

To become hypnotized, you will have to follow all of your doctor's suggestions. He may begin by asking you to stare at an imaginary spot on the ceiling directly above your forehead. (left)

When your eyelids become heavy and you find it difficult to keep them open, you are well on your way toward hypnosis. (right)

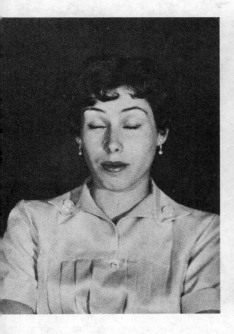 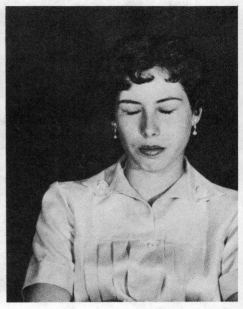

At your doctor's suggestion, you will find it almost impossible to open your eyes. No matter how hard you try, as long as you want to go deeper relaxed, you will not be able to open them. (left)

After a short while you'll stop trying to open your eyes and just let yourself go completely relaxed. This is the first stage of hypnosis. (right)

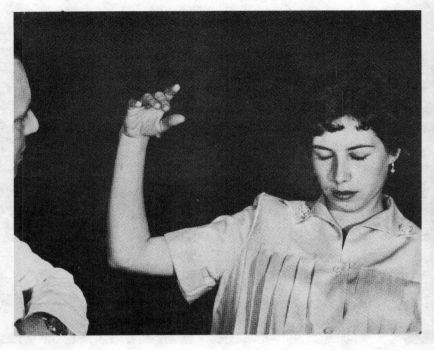

To go still deeper relaxed, your doctor will say, you need only let your arm rise slowly upward.

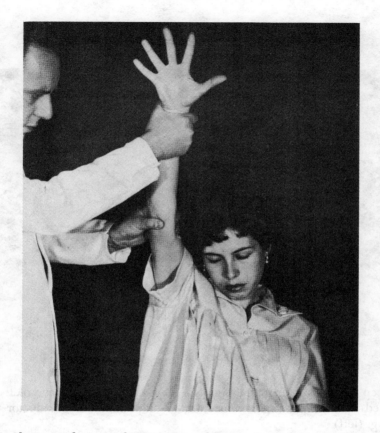

In the second, or cataleptic, stage of hypnosis, your arm will become stiff and rigid. Your doctor will not be able to bend it (only you can, if you really wish to) and you can keep it in that position for a long time without tiring.

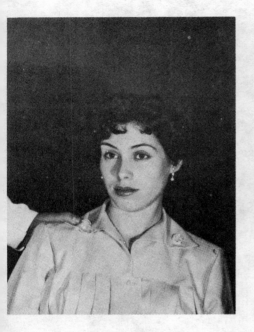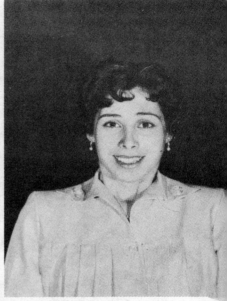

Deep hypnosis (the somnambulistic stage) will find you completely relaxed with your thoughts concentrated only on what your doctor is saying. (left)

After your hypnosis, at your doctor's suggestion, you will dehypnotize or "alert" yourself within a few seconds. You will feel refreshed—as if you have just awakened from a good night's comfortable sleep. (right)

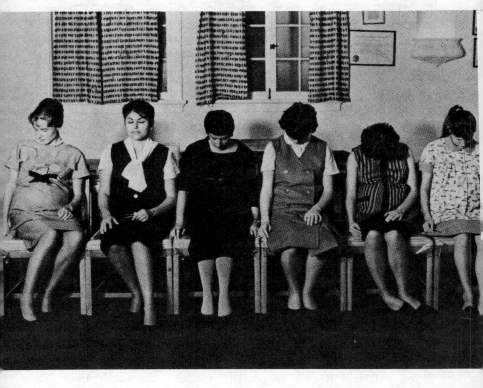

Group training classes in hypnosis, with other pregnant women, will be an important part of your preparations for a comfortable delivery.

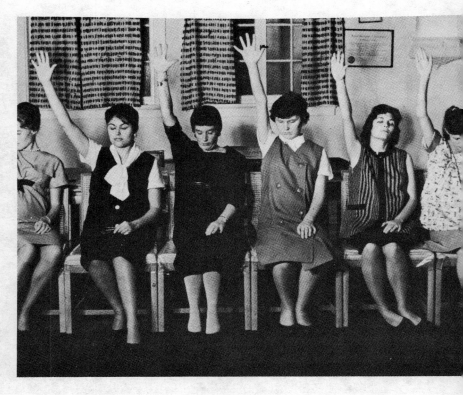

You will find it easy to practice reaching the cataleptic stage of hypnosis in the company of these other women.

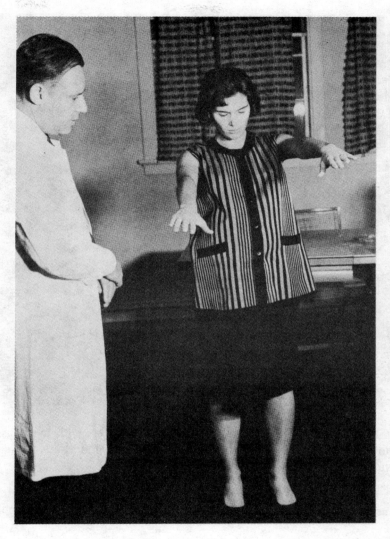

Sometimes your doctor will want to find out how susceptible you are to hypnosis before he starts your formal training.
He may give you a "susceptibility test" which involves your
imagining that you have a heavy bucket of water on the
back of one outstretched hand.

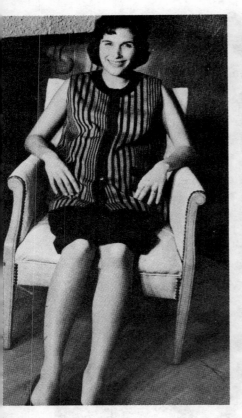 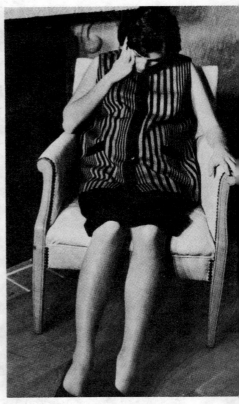

Practice alone at home is essential to your success with hypnosis. To do this you will need no special "props"; only a comfortable chair in a quiet room for a few minutes each day. (left)

In these home sessions you will practice making one hand numb and insensitive to pain. This is the start of "glove anesthesia" with hypnosis. (right)

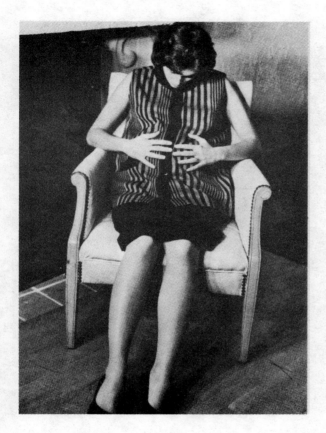

Glove anesthesia, you will learn, may be transferred from the hand to any part of your body—such as the abdomen—merely by touching your hand to that part.

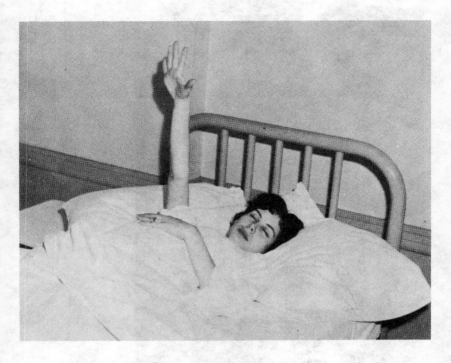

The outstretched hand as a sign of deeper hypnosis will show your doctor the progress you are making toward relaxation after you arrive at the hospital.

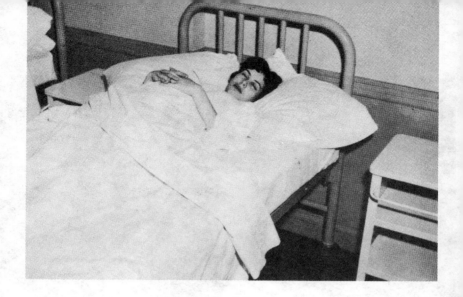

Active labor with hypnosis will be an exciting experience. You will be aware of your contractions, but you will not feel the pain commonly associated with them.

You may, if you wish, feel what it is like to be in active labor without hypnosis. Then you can be speedily rehypnotized.

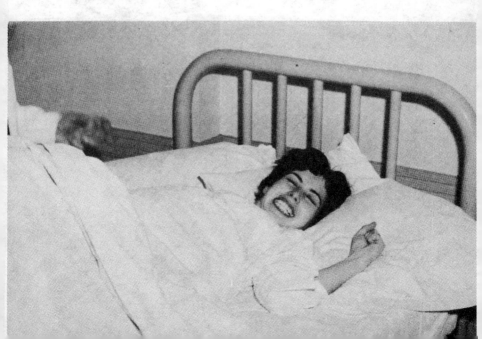

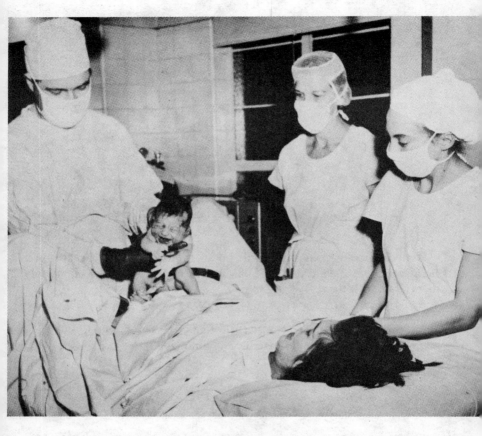

Your first glimpse of your baby, at the moment of birth, will be the most rewarding experience of your life—the fulfillment of your role as a mother.

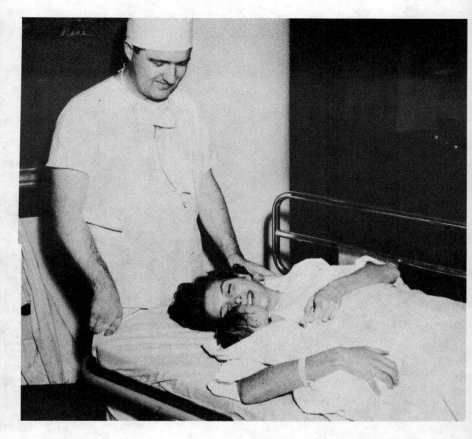

Tender loving care, an emotional experience which your infant senses very early in life, begins with that first meeting in the delivery room. Hypnosis can help make this moment one you'll both experience with profound peace.

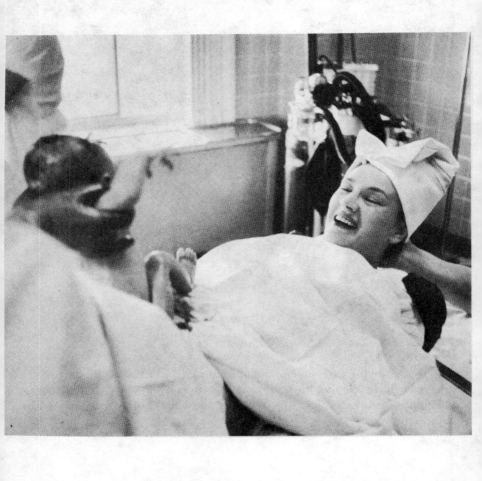

Childbirth with Hypnosis

·

by WILLIAM S. KROGER, M. D.

edited by JULES STEINBERG

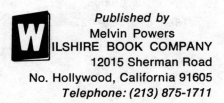

Published by
Melvin Powers
WILSHIRE BOOK COMPANY
12015 Sherman Road
No. Hollywood, California 91605
Telephone: (213) 875-1711

Wilshire Book Company edition
is published by special arrangement
with Doubleday & Company, Inc., New York

Printed by

HAL LEIGHTON PRINTING COMPANY
P.O. Box 3952
North Hollywood, California 91605
Telephone: (213) 983-1105

PHOTOGRAPHS COURTESY OF

THE CHICAGO MEDICAL SCHOOL
THE DEPARTMENT OF PHOTOGRAPHY
(PHOTOGRAPHER: T. SCANLAN)

QUEEN OF ANGELS HOSPITAL,
LOS ANGELES, CALIFORNIA

LIFE AND STAN WAYMAN,
COPYRIGHT © 1958 BY TIME, INC.

To *Jimmy Louise and Janet,* our wives,
whose constant attendance at the birth
of this volume helped, materially,
to ease the authors' labors.

CONTENTS

INTRODUCTION

OBSTETRICS AND HYPNOSIS are two of the oldest departments of medicine. Many references to the art of midwifery are to be found in the Old Testament and the earlier scriptures of ancient Egypt. In fact, one such papyrus, which Egyptologists tell us was written in the year 1553 B.C., prescribes a potion of sea salts and grains plastered on the abdomen to delay the onset of labor. To hasten delivery, this early obstetrician suggests a stinging application of peppermint to the "posterior" of the patient.

Despite this interest of pre-Christian Era man in applied medicine—and a surprisingly large number of his home-brewed remedies and devices for alleviating some of the discomforts of childbirth are still employed in Oriental countries—all disease and suffering of that time were ascribed to capricious gods, whose whimsies, it was thought, were understood only by the priests.

Asa, king of Judah, is censured in the second book of the Chronicles (16:12) for turning not to the Lord, but to the physicians, to cure the disease in his feet which afflicted him in the thirty-ninth year of his reign. (As if to oblige his critics, Asa succumbed to his illness two years later.) In Egypt, meanwhile, fifteen centuries before the birth of Christ, the god Sekhem was thought to be the protector of a mother in childbirth.

With the health of the populace thus blindly entrusted to the priests, numerous methods for appeasing the wrath of the gods were recorded. These ranged from the "sleep temples" of the Egyptians to the divine "laying on of hands" popular with the desert tribes. In the days of the Greek domination of civilization, the physically or mentally ill were placed in hypnotic-like states by the oracles and priests for healing by the "God of Medicine." Of course, the cures obtained then were not attributed to hypnosis. (The word itself, which is a misnomer derived from the Greek "hypnos," meaning sleep, was not coined until the middle of the nineteenth century.) Instead, the results were attributed to miracles performed by the gods.

This notion that all illness and cure were the result of divine providence persisted for nearly three thousand years. For the longest period, the pains of labor were thought to be an inescapable consequence of bringing a new creature, cursed with original sin, into the world. The penalty for tampering with this divine justice through pain-relieving measures, even in those countries which had begun to emerge from the Dark Ages, was extreme.

In 1591, according to court records in the city of Edinburgh, Scotland, one Eufame MacLayne was duly tried and convicted of a most serious crime. Apparently the defendant, a young mother of twin babies, had committed the offense of requesting an analgesic drug for her labors from the midwife who attended the birth of her children. This, the record states, was "contrary to divine law and in contempt of the Crown." For this futile attempt to break with the superstitions of her day, Eufame paid with her life by burning at the stake.

The next one hundred fifty years or so were marked by humanity's fierce struggle to help itself, despite the restraints of religious dogma. Many martyrs were consumed in the fires fanned by ignorance and fear, but gradually the taboos of thousands of years' standing were whittled away. By the end of the eighteenth century, the atmosphere was such that a theory of "animal magnetism," developed by a Viennese physician, Anton Mesmer, had won popular approval throughout Europe.

Mesmer, whose principles are erroneously supposed by

many persons to be the forerunner of modern hypnotic procedures, contended that the ability of one individual to relieve the pain of another was derived from certain magnetic forces originating in astral bodies. However, he imparted his curative powers through a touch of his hand or a "magnetized" rod in a dimly lit, perfumed room with mysterious-sounding background music. With such props he effected a surprisingly large number of cures.

For a while the doctor from Vienna had more patients than he could handle. His popularity extended even to the French court of Louis XVI. Finally, though, as must happen to all fads, the sleigh ride came to a bumpy end. Egged on by contemporary physicians, a commission of the French government branded Mesmer a fraud, and mesmerism as a form of therapy fell into disrepute.

Still, the seed of a new medical concept had been planted. The idea of suggestive therapy, or the ability of a patient to help himself to get well simply by expecting relief, captured the imaginations of a handful of doctors of the day. Experiments along more scientific lines, particularly with the control of painful sensations, continued.

By the mid-1800s, a British practitioner, Dr. James Braid, had refined Mesmer's crude trappings to the point where he could induce an air of expectancy in many patients simply by having them stare at a bright object. Braid, who wrote many scientific papers on the subject, was the first to apply the term "hypnosis" to the procedure.

While many physicians of that day stood fast in their opposition to any new technique, others continued the research where Braid left off. One of his disciples, Dr. James Esdaile, practicing in India, performed over three hundred major operations (including limb amputations and the surgical removal of tumors) with no other anesthetic than hypnosis. In France, England, and the United States other physicians began to employ the new method, often risking professional censure in their search for a more effective and less harmful pain-relieving agent.

All this while, the practice of obstetrics also continued its slow but steady rise from the pit of ignorance to which thousands of superstition-filled years had consigned it. For example, the method of using obstetrical forceps to facilitate delivery of women in difficult labor was first discovered around the middle of the sixteenth century. However, even this boon was to be denied women for three generations thereafter while the Chamberlens, a family of physicians, attempted to pass the secret from father to son in order to squeeze the last ounce of profit out of the discovery. But news of the use of forceps did leak out, and many great medical pioneers lent their geniuses to the further development of this important instrument.

The Hungarian doctor Ignaz Philipp Semmelweis's conquest of childbed fever, the Frenchman Karl Franz Credé's successful campaign against blindness in newborn infants, and the British physician Joseph Lister's work in antiseptic surgery were combined with the work of other noble scientists to make childbirth the almost completely safe procedure that it is today for both mother and child.

Sad to relate, though, each step of the way was fought against the rear-guard actions of obstetricians who preferred to maintain the status quo rather than give way to progress. Opposition to Semmelweis's theory that he could materially reduce the number of deaths in maternity cases by the simple expedient of having those in the delivery room wash their hands in an antiseptic solution was so great that the discoverer brooded himself into insanity attempting to answer the attacks upon him.

Introduction

The first physicians to use hypnosis as a tool in their medical armamentarium found both the public and the profession no less critical of their methods. Indeed, the period from the denunciation of Mesmer to the mid-twentieth century was marked by many splits among doctors themselves over the therapeutic value of simple suggestion and other hypnotic procedures. Oddly enough, both those who thought too little of hypnosis and those who expected too much of the medium were responsible for keeping the public confused for hundreds of years. The former thought that hypnosis was, at best, a trick of the stage magician, while the latter thought that hypnosis could do anything from removing warts to curing serious illnesses.

Those firm "believers" did achieve some measure of success with cures for a few diseases which, today, we know as being psychosomatic in origin, or resulting from a subconscious wish to be ill. Their results, on the other hand, did not warrant the blind faith that some persons placed in hypnosis or in hypnosis-based religions—only to condemn the entire procedure when it failed to live up to their expectations.

One of the physicians who appreciated the value of hypnosis early in its development was the eminent French doctor, Hyppolite Bernheim, who abandoned his tradition-bound medical practice to conduct research on hypnotic therapeutics exclusively. Around the end of the nineteenth century he founded the Nancy (France) School of Hypnotism. It was there that one of Bernheim's students, Dr. Sigmund Freud, worked out his now famous theories of psychoanalysis.

Freud readily admitted that many of his penetrating insights into the workings of the mind came about because of his interest in hypnosis. For instance, one of the experiments which he witnessed at the Nancy school concerned the overcoming of posthypnotic amnesia, the inability of the subject to remember anything that had transpired during hypnosis. The eager student, Freud, observed how, when the subject was urged to make an effort to recall what had been said to him, he eventually remembered everything. This lesson led directly to Freud's development of the "free association" method of analysis, which evolved into the psychoanalysis we know today.

Regrettably, though, Freud was a poor hypnotist, judging by present-day standards, and so hypnosis played only a minor role in his later work. By his own accounts, Freud was baffled by hypnotic phenomena, which he knew were objective but which he was never able to explain in the light of his own theories. We can only guess how far this genius would have taken us had he known about our newest techniques of self-conditioning with hypnosis or about the more recent understanding that the hypnotic state is *not* a sleep state and is not even remotely related to unconsciousness. For, even without the knowledge of these advances, Freud stated that psychoanalysis has merely inherited the estate left by hypnosis.

But while the popularity of psychoanalysis eclipsed that of hypnosis for a short time and the subject of suggestion was barred from many serious medical discussions, a handful of scientists continued to battle popular confusion and misunderstanding of the true goals of hypnosis. One of these men, Pierre Janet, the great French psychologist who first opposed hypnosis and later advocated its use, observed: "If my work is not ready today, it will be tomorrow, when there will be a new turn to Fashion's wheel which will bring back hypnotism as surely as our grandmothers' styles."

And so it has! Hypnotism is more popular with physicians

and patients alike than ever before. The subject is on the curriculum of many reputable colleges and medical schools; its use in controlling the pain and fear of drilling and injection and in suppressing gagging tendencies is an established procedure in thousands of dental practices; and in 1958 the American Medical Association, charged with maintaining the professional standards of doctors in this country, placed its qualified stamp of approval on the medical use of hypnosis.

"The use of hypnosis has a recognized place in the medical armamentarium," the A.M.A. stated, "and is a useful technique in the treatment of certain illnesses, when employed by qualified medical personnel."

Three years earlier, the British Medical Association, in endorsing the procedure under that country's National Health Service program, stated: "In suitable subjects, it [hypnosis] is an effective method of relieving pain in childbirth without altering the normal course of labour."

In this country no one person has contributed more to the development of suggestive procedures to mitigate childbirth pain than Dr. Joseph B. DeLee. He was among the first to express the opinion that a woman in labor need have no more pain than she is willing to bear, and he recognized, over twenty years ago, that with hypnosis some patients could relax profoundly during delivery. Dr. DeLee advocated hypnosis as being the "only anesthetic without danger" and told the profession: "I am irked when I see my colleagues neglect to avail themselves of this harmless and potent remedy."

Thanks to the efforts of Dr. DeLee and others, a pregnant woman today who wishes to deliver her child with the aid of suggestion and/or hypnosis will find little difficulty in locating a physician schooled in the use of this not so mysterious procedure. In part, *Childbirth with Hypnosis*, inspired by the tireless research of such men, is intended as a guide to what the patient/subject might expect in the doctor's office and the hospital delivery room. But this book is not calculated to appeal primarily to the faddist or attention-seeker who will try this procedure or that remedy simply because she will be the first of her crowd to do so.

Today's better-educated patient wants to know and deserves to be told everything that science is doing to protect her health and that of her child during childbirth. We no longer burn women at the stake for seeking pain-relieving measures. If the modern patient is wise, she will seek competent medical advice; but she will also demand all of the facts, not evasive answers or old wives' tales. Shorn of its mysticism in this healthy atmosphere, hypnosis cannot fail to thrive. In fact, one of the aims of hypnosis when it is used in childbirth is to remove, as much as possible, the superstitions and malicious gossip which have surrounded pregnancy and labor ever since the back-yard fence was invented.

In this volume, too, we have attempted to take much of the mystery out of hypnosis. The reader will find frank discussions of the background, technique, and advantages of each of the common phenomena of hypnosis, including those few which can only be described as "unexplainable." We believe that we have played entirely fair with both the profession and the expectant mother by adhering to this scientific approach of admitting what we do not know. The patient who needs it does not, after all, refuse to accept beneficial brain surgery simply because the surgeon cannot scientifically account for the origin of the spark of life.

The manner in which hypnosis can help alleviate the fear, tension, and pain of childbirth, however, will call for no such charity from the reader. We shall state, positively, that hypnosis contains none of the supernatural aspects ascribed to it by our ancestors. It is, we shall demonstrate, the most natural state imaginable, deriving its health-stimulating powers from the self-concentration, or self-discipline if you will, of the subject.

This is not to imply that *Childbirth with Hypnosis* is intended to be a how-to-do-it book for amateur hypnotists. That would be as foolish as insisting that any other facet of medicine can be learned just by reading one book on the subject. The professional approach to hypnosis is just as important. Unleashing a subject's reservoir of mental and physical strength, with hypnosis, carries a responsibility which the physician alone is best trained to bear.

But patients, too, have an obligation. They owe it to themselves, as well as to their unborn children, to leave no page unturned in their quest for safe, comfortable child-birth.

WILLIAM S. KROGER, M.D.

9735 WILSHIRE BOULEVARD
BEVERLY HILLS, CALIFORNIA

CHAPTER I

•

Childbirth—
The Fulfillment

YOU WILL KNOW when your baby is ready to be born.

Whether or not you are going to deliver with the assistance of hypnosis, the beginnings of your labor will be marked by a slight discomfort in the back. You will feel these rhythmic contractions—or labor pains, as they are often mistakenly called—as a tightening of the uterus, a hardening of your entire abdomen. Very likely you will have experienced these sensations as irregularly-spaced contractions on and off throughout the last month of your pregnancy.

The twingelike feelings of true labor, however, will be fairly evenly spaced—at first, perhaps, as much as twenty minutes apart. At the onset, too, these twinges will build up in intensity and then disappear completely, often within thirty seconds. But, as your labor progresses, the contractions will last longer, up to a minute or so, and will come closer together. At this time, there may also be a passing of a small amount of blood-tinged mucus and a gushing of fluid from the vagina.

These symptoms, singularly or together, mark the onset of labor. They are certainly no cause for fear or anxiety. On the contrary, as you will discover for yourself, your months of prenatal training in hypnosis and education about childbirth will have taught you exactly how to relax and how to face the next few hours confidently—dimly aware of slight discomforts and minor irritations, but with every fiber of your mind and body concentrated on the happy fulfillment of your feminine role. *At no time will you experience more pain than you are willing to bear.*

Your physician—and at this point you should be in communication with him—will advise you when to leave for the hospital. If you are hypnotically oriented, he may even attempt to relax you further by suggesting relaxation to you over the telephone. In any event, no matter how deeply relaxed you may become, you will continue to feel the contractions, time the interval between twinges, and relay this information to your doctor.

Perhaps a word is in order here about a condition popularly known as "false labor." These are contractions, not unlike true labor, which are sometimes present just before a patient reaches full term. They are frequently observed in those women whose desire to "get it over with" is more pronounced than normal. Yet, while the intensity of this "false labor" may even surpass that of the genuine type, it can be identified by its irregularity and its failure to increase in severity as time goes on.

It is important that you, as an expectant mother, realize that these "false" pains are neither exaggerated nor imaginary. They may logically result when, prior to the commencement of your actual labor, your uterus slowly engages the baby's head into the pelvis. Then, too, from what we shall learn of the nature of pain in the following chapters, it will be obvious that anxiousness over the birth of your child can be reflected in the sympathetic nervous system's causing tensions and consequent contractions of the muscle fibers around the uterus. Certainly fewer of these false starts are to be seen among self-controlled, relaxed mothers-to-be.

The purpose of true labor, naturally, is to permit easy physical passage of your baby through the gradually expanding birth canal. As a first step, it is necessary for the neck of the uterus, which is called the cervix, to widen sufficiently for the baby to pass through. Your body accomplishes this by contractions of the uterine muscle. Normally, this is an involuntary act over which you will have no control. This is similar to the actions of the muscles around the intestines or the heart which tend to perform their functions at a predetermined rate. The length of time for this phase of labor, therefore, will not necessarily be the same for you as it is for other women; nor will it be the same for your second or third child as it was for your first.

On the average, women with first babies spend approximately sixteen hours in labor, from the first labor pain to the delivery of the afterbirth. With subsequent children, the neck of the uterus, as well as the vagina, will be less resistant to dilatation, and consequently the duration of labor may be ten hours or less. No one can state for certain how long your labor will last once it starts. Much will depend upon your physical condition and your emotional attitude at the time. Still, there is very real evidence to support the theory that a more relaxed state can effect the onset of labor.

A survey of some 1,000 typical confinements at a Chicago hospital with which the author was affiliated reveals that in 306 cases labor began sometime between midnight and 6 A.M., hours when the patients were most truly at rest. Only 182 women started their contractions between the busier hours of noon and 6 P.M., and commencement of the remaining childbirths was evenly scattered throughout the day.

No matter when you labor begins, however, the importance of relaxing throughout the first stage cannot be overstated. It is too simple a matter for the tensions of the moment, magnified perhaps by such actions as the clenching of fists or writhing around on the bed, to make the contractions appear more severe than they really are.

Later you will discover how and why hypnosis can help you to achieve control over your discomforts. We need only state here that in biweekly office visits and group training classes, beginning around the sixth month of your pregnancy, you will learn how to relax all of your muscles and to breathe slowly and deeply when you feel a contraction commencing.

When you finally arrive at the hospital, these contractions will be spaced about fifteen or twenty minutes apart. After the customary admitting routine—and no matter how relaxed you might be, you will be fully aware of the questions the attendants ask—preparations for your baby's delivery will begin.

Depending upon the practices of the institution and the wishes of your physician, these preparations can involve shaving the hairs around your genitals and giving you an enema. Prior to this, in almost all hospitals, your medical history will have been recorded and an examination made to determine just how far the cervix has opened and how far into the pelvis the baby's head has descended.

All this while, the relaxing techniques you will have learned should keep you comfortable and free from fear or anxiety. Your physician may, at this time, elect to induce a deeper hypnotic state by using any one of a number of methods similar to those mentioned in Chapter III. He will advise you to relax continuously and to hear only the suggestions of the person whom both of you will have selected for deepening your hypnosis. This is known as the transfer of hypnotic rapport.

There is an increasing tendency among physicians and hospital officials to permit the husband to remain with the patient throughout this phase of labor. Your husband's presence will be particularly advisable if he has attended your classes in the elementary lessons of hypnosis and if, through your physician, he has been placed in hypnotic rapport with you so that he can reinforce the suggestions of relaxation. In this manner, rather than feeling frustratingly useless, your husband can assume an active role in the proceedings. But it is not vital that he be at hand, because hypnotic rapport may be transferred easily from your doctor to a staff physician or nurse.

The second stage of your labor, especially if it is rapid, may require that you be taken to the hospital's delivery room. This section of the delivery lasts from the time the cervix is fully opened until delivery of the infant. (The third stage of labor is that period from the birth of the baby to delivery of the afterbirth or placenta.) Your baby's head has now passed through the uterine mouth into the vagina. The backache that you have been feeling may be gone, but the final stretching of the uterus can produce sharp discomfort. This "pain" need not be cause for alarm because it, too, will vanish after some ten or more contractions.

Here, as at any stage in your delivery, you may feel what it is like to go through your labor unaided by hypnosis. Many women want to experience fully a "pain" or two, because hypnosis is such an uncomplicated affair that they cannot honestly believe that it helps. Other women feel that some pain is part of the over-all pattern of childbirth. They would be missing a part of this rich experience, they believe, if they did not feel at least one undiluted pain.

Your physician will have arranged a simple signal for alerting you from the hypnotic state. If you wish it, he can terminate your hypnosis merely by touching you on one shoulder. Just as simply, he can reinduce hypnosis by touching you on the other shoulder or by using some other signal upon which both of you will have agreed; or you may have been trained to induce self-hypnosis and to dehypnotize yourself at will.

In any case, the hypnosis will *not* inhibit the progress of your labor. After a brief interval, to permit sufficient rotation and descent of your infant's head, you will feel a rectal pressure very much the same as the sensation when a large movement needs to be passed. This will be the distended vagina pressing against the rectum, a feeling which will remain with you until your baby is born.

The sensations in your pelvis now are being felt both as distentions in the vagina and pressure at the rectum. When these begin, you will be instructed to take a deep breath slowly with your mouth closed, holding it tightly shut until the contraction has reached its greatest strength. Then you will take second, third, and fourth breaths, while pushing down on the rectum, for as long as the uterine contraction lasts.

With each of these contractions, you will push down as if you are straining to have a bowel movement. This will not be difficult. In fact, it will seem to be a most natural response to the pressures in your pelvic regions. The important thing to remember is that you must relax between, not during, these contractions.

All this while, as specific physical changes take place within your body, you will pass through certain emotional phases directly connected with the progress of your labor. These reactions are common to almost all women in childbirth, and they respond very well to the relaxing procedures of hypnosis which you will have mastered.

In the first place, if you are like most other women, you will be intently relieved by the realization that you are really doing something to assist in the birth of your baby. The well-being of the infant will be your primary consideration. During the periods between contractions, you will gradually lose more of your conscious awareness of what is going on around you. The artificial social world in which we all live will disappear as labor progresses, until you are saying things and speaking in a language form totally unlike your normal self.

Then, at some point during the pressure and stretching, just before the baby's head makes its appearance, you may be seized by a momentary fear that not enough progress is being made. This, too, is fairly typical, although one of the aims of hypnosis is to control such fears so that you, the patient, will experience a minimum of discomfort and will continue to assist the contractions. Still, it is not unusual for women, especially those with no training in hypnosis, to demand chemical anesthesia at this time. Presently we shall have more to say about the all-important subject of this type of anesthesia.

Failure to assist the contractions often produces more discomfort than normal; usually, the pain is not extreme. This you must sincerely believe, and if you have any doubts, they should be resolved before you reach the end of your pregnancy. Even the afore-mentioned emotional reaction of fear soon gives way to the relaxed state noted in earlier labor. Very quickly you will, again, think only of the welfare of your baby.

We have observed that if a woman at this stage notices the physicians and nurses around her at all, it is only to apologize for the trouble she thinks she has caused. This, we might add, is certainly unnecessary, because these trained individuals know that such emotional responses of a woman to childbirth are as natural as the birth process itself.

Returning to the subject of anesthesia, it is important

that we correct a common misconception of the use of hypnosis in childbirth. Drugs and chemical anesthetics are always available for labor, as well as in the delivery room, should a woman want them or should they be needed. *Hypnosis never precludes the administration of drugs.* We never solicit any promise from patients that they will refrain from asking for anesthesia; nor do we consider it a breach of confidence for them to do so. The truth of the matter is that less than ten per cent of the women can go through the entire course of labor and delivery of their babies without some chemical assistance.

The amount of assistance required will vary with a number of factors, not the least important of which is how much the physician considers can be safely administered without endangering the health of the mother and child. Recent medical research indicates that when excessive "knockout" drugs are given for the relief of pain without regard to the health of the child, the oxygen supply to the fetus may be decreased.

Passing from the mother's blood stream into the placental circulation, these respiratory-depressing drugs may even cut down on the amount of the oxygen flow to the fetus, necessitating resuscitation after birth. There is, apparently, considerable evidence to support the theory that some cases of mental retardation, cerebral palsy, epilepsy, and other brain diseases in infants are due to this condition, known as fetal anoxia.

What is probably best, at least from the point of view of assisting the greatest number of women, is a combination of hypnosis and local infiltration (novocain). The latter form of anesthesia gives pain relief similar to that afforded by the injection your dentist gives. The combination is a near perfect prescription for painless childbirth, as it is safe and sure in its action. Hypnosis can be used with chemical forms of anesthesia, such as gas, ether, or drugs. This method of pain relief is known as hypnonarcosis. It offers women the satisfying, relaxing experience of hypnosis with a minimum amount of sleep-inducing drugs. Most patients remain in some degree of hypnosis during most of their labor and delivery, and only a small dosage of drugs is required to "take the edge off" the pains.

During those moments just before the birth of your child, your pelvic and abdominal muscles will have eased the baby down through the birth canal. Each time you bear down, the baby will descend farther toward the outlet of the vagina, which distends its walls until there is sufficient room for the head and body to pass through.

Perhaps you are one of those women who become dismayed at the thought of the vagina distending enough for the passage of the child. You might even have heard that deep tears are inevitable in the process of childbirth. This is positively not true. Nature has spent nine months preparing this outlet for the stretching and for the delivery of your baby through the entire length of the birth canal. The chances are excellent that the passage will be achieved without any abnormal resistance from the walls of the vagina.

In most cases—particularly in those women having their first child—where the opening is not naturally large enough, it is quite customary for the physician to make a short incision called an episiotomy. Both this incision and its subsequent repair are relatively minor procedures, usually performed while the patient is under the influence of a local anesthetic. In any event, there is little or no discomfort. It is even possible, in those limited cases where a woman has reached a truly deep state of hypnosis, for the doctor to manage this operation without recourse to chemical anesthesia.

Now the stage is set for enactment of the final scene in the drama of the birth of your child. In those final moments, just before the head of your infant appears, you may pass through yet another emotional phase. This will be marked by a sensation of burning around the lips of the vagina and by a feeling that you are about to burst open. There will even be a tendency to resist your final contractions, but your attention will not be diverted for long from the task at hand.

You will concentrate upon the suggestion of your physician to push down "real hard" as if your bowels are going to move. It is at this point that the head of your infant may emerge without your being aware of it. The next contraction will free the shoulders and may even expel the entire body of the child. This will be greeted with an emotion which you, as a new mother, will never have experienced before, and which you will never forget.

With the very first cry of your new baby, you will be overwhelmed with pride and satisfaction in your achievement. You will forget, for the moment, all the painful sensations of your labor. Women who are awake at this time report that their minds are entirely possessed by the child. There is no greater joy, they say, than when, after the umbilical cord has been painlessly severed, the infant is handed to them.

What better way is there to cap the experience we have just described than to quote the words of a woman who has delivered her infant with the assistance of hypnosis? Mrs. S.L., a young mother whose first child was delivered in a Midwestern hospital, writes: "My labor pains started about midnight on Sunday. I immediately thought of the many sessions I had with my doctor and fellow patients, and could feel only a little apprehension mixed with a great deal of excitement. As my labor progressed, I remembered all of the 'relaxation methods' I'd been taught.

"At the hospital, my contractions came closer together. But, after my doctor hypnotized me, I became still much more relaxed. I was even more aware of my contractions, but they were in no way uncomfortable. As a matter of fact, I was so relaxed that I went into a light sleep between the contractions.

"The doctor allowed my husband to stay in the labor room with me. He [the husband] would help to remind me to stay under hypnosis. Even though it took until 11:00 A.M. the next morning before I was ready for the second stage of labor, I was still not too tired, and felt quite relaxed.

"In the delivery room, my contractions came quite rapidly. I panted with the contractions, and concentrated on relaxing while they went away. My doctor spoke to me often. I went a little deeper under hypnosis with each of his words. Still, I was completely conscious of what was going on. The anesthesiologist was standing right beside me, but so far we did not feel any urgent need for anything he could offer.

"Then, the baby's head was emerging. I felt tremendous pressure, and was lifted up to see the baby's head coming out. It was really a unique experience: one which I shall never forget. My doctor told me that it was a boy. I opened my eyes wide, to see a pink baby, wriggling and crying without any need to be slapped. He was an extremely healthy boy!

"My recovery was fast and without any complications. Except for the episiotomy, for which I was given a 'shot' of novocain locally, I did not have any anesthetic. I am now expecting another baby. I intend to have this one the same way."

Essentially, then, this is natural childbirth. We need not concern ourselves here with such matters as the third, or placental, stage of labor. This is a painless expulsion of the afterbirth that takes place anywhere up to fifteen minutes after delivery. Following the birth of your child, it will be an anti-climax, and it will have no bearing upon your emotional state as a mother.

Types of delivery

Natural, normal delivery, with or without hypnosis, is the safest type of delivery. It is also the most rewarding experience for the mother. Unfortunately, however, not all babies are delivered in the manner we have been describing. The number of Caesarean sections, for example, has been increasing each year until, at present, about one out of fifty infants in the United States is born via this procedure.

This type of delivery involves major surgery through the abdominal wall and uterus. After the child has been removed through these openings, the incisions are repaired by stitching. There are, of course, several purely physical reasons for delivering a child by Caesarean section. The mother's pelvis may be so unusually small that it will impede the passage of the baby. Still more rarely, the afterbirth may have separated from the uterine wall or attached itself to a part of the uterus in front of the baby's head. Such uncommon occurrences may prompt the physician to consider a Caesarean section. On the other hand, many women insist upon this type of delivery although there is little physical evidence to justify the decision.

Very likely, it is the prospect of bypassing what she considers to be painful labor which prompts the less mature woman even to think of giving up her child in a Caesarean birth. The operation is surely as safe as any modern surgical procedure. Still, it deprives the mother of the sense of fulfillment which comes from participating fully in the birth of her child. Furthermore, most physicians consider that the scar on the uterus makes it inadvisable for these women ever again to bear children except via Caesarean section. This price, well-adjusted women agree, is too great to pay to satisfy easily controlled fears and anxieties.

Another term that a woman might encounter in discussions of difficulty in childbearing is the "breech" method of delivery. This is a type of birth where the buttocks and feet of the infant emerge first and the head afterwards. Provided that the mother's pelvic measurements are adequate, this manner of delivery will be no more distressing than a normal birth.

It is a purely physical phenomenon that some infants (less than three per cent of those born each year) who may be in the breech position during pregnancy fail to change this position before labor starts. The birth of these babies carries a somewhat greater strain for the physician and some minute element of danger for the child. But, contrary to the situation which existed just a generation ago, such deliveries are not a major obstetrical problem. They should not be cause for anxiety on the part of the mother.

A third technique of delivery under less than usual circumstances that has been vastly improved over the past twenty or twenty-five years is the method of forceps delivery. This is commonly referred to as "taking the baby with instruments." It involves the use of obstetrical forceps, or two separate S-shaped blades with smooth, curved inner surfaces.

In an otherwise perfectly normal birth, it may become advisable for the doctor to assist the baby through the vaginal outlet by means of this instrument, especially if it is the first-born. The blades fit snugly against the infant's head, and the physician's gentle traction on the handles completes the delivery. It is a simple procedure. As far as she is concerned, the mother is merely relieved of the final fifteen minutes or so of labor. However, the decision to use the forceps is determined by purely physical factors present at the time of birth.

The post-partum period

The period immediately following delivery and lasting from six to eight weeks is known as the post-partum period or the puerperium. It is a time for certain physical changes which return a mother's body to its pre-pregnant state. Also, during this time, emotional patterns are established, and they can affect a woman's happiness in her new role, as well as alter the psychological development of her child.

For some six days following the birth of your child, your activities will be closely supervised and you will be obliged to adhere to a tightly regimented program. It is extremely unlikely that you will feel anything but fine. The only real danger, therefore, is that you may overdo your activities in your haste to return to a normal way of life.

During the post-partum period, it is important that nothing interferes with either the return of the stretched birth canal to its natural shape or the regaining of tone of the muscles around the uterus. This is vital to prevent sagging of the pelvic organs. In addition, the separation of the placenta from the wall of the uterus during the third stage of labor leaves a very real wound, which the new mother may recognize as a sore spot. To avoid the possibility of internal bleeding or infection, the large blood vessels in this area must be permitted to heal. Time, and time alone, is the great healer. With just a little bit of patience, almost all new mothers are soon "as good as new"—physically speaking, that is.

Psychologically, your adjustment to your new role can be just as simple, although, to be perfectly candid, it is less understood. It is certainly normal to expect that you will be a bit apprehensive of your ability to care properly for the little newcomer. The skills of motherhood are not, after all, automatically acquired with the birth of the child. Yet the likelihood remains that this overconcern will be mixed with an "emotional lag" resulting from the intense build-up of a feeling of motherliness during pregnancy.

You may detect an inclination on your part, after the initial excitement of childbirth has passed, to look upon your small child and wonder: "Is this all there is to it?" Many mothers can recall the empty feeling they had at this time, and they remember how they compensated for it by dwelling upon pleasurable fantasies of pregnancy.

If you experience them at all, these "blue" periods last but a few days, and they end abruptly in your rapidly adapting to your new role as a mother. The important factor in this adjustment will be your way of experiencing the demands made on you by the infant. To put it another way, as a new mother you must maintain a healthy attitude towards learning to meet these demands. In this connection, you will find the discipline of self-hypnosis helpful in increasing your ability to learn new things.

The woman who fails to take motherhood in stride may exhibit her maladjustment in many ways ranging from extreme concern to marked indifference or actual neglect. She will attempt to flee from the responsibilities of her new status by delegating her child's care to a nurse. The "bottle propper" who refuses even to hold her infant while nursing is another typical example. Finally, we are all familiar with the case of the mother who tries to resolve her emotional conflicts by displaying some physical symptom which, she hopes, will square her neglectful behavior in the eyes of her family and friends. "Poor Mary," they'll say. "Those horrible headaches are preventing her from taking care of her baby."

Truly, these are instances of abnormal behavior. Your own "letdown" feeling, coming on the heels of childbirth, need not end in such extreme actions. It will help considerably if you will discuss your fears and anxieties frankly, with yourself first, and then with someone in whom you have a great deal of confidence. The choking down of emotions at this time will only create further tensions when you can least afford them.

Infant psychology

The effect upon the infant of unconscious rejection, or even hesitation, on the part of the mother is something else again. Doctors and psychologists now accept the fact that even newborn babies are quite capable of "feeling" such emotions as anger, frustration, and fear. They recognize, too, a certain "emotional contagion," wherein the uncertainties and doubts of the mother are transmitted to the child. If, for example, the mother is not certain that she really wants the baby, the infant can usually sense it.

At present we can only guess about the full impact of these factors on the psychological and physical development of the child. The very latest medical research shows that when the emotional needs of the infant are denied, we may expect a higher percentage of gastric ulcers, colitis, obesity, and other nervous ailments in later life. Psychoanalysts, too, are quite familiar with the pattern of adult insecurity and anxiety arising from inadequate satisfaction of the infant's needs.

During the first two years or so of your child's life, his requirements will be quite simple. You will easily recognize the need for food, evacuation, warmth, and freedom from such irritations as sticking diaper pins. All babies require these things, but in the case of the first two there is an element of timing which makes each infant an individual according to his own physical make-up. When these individual traits are ignored, as in the instance of too rigid or too early toilet training or fixed feeding times, the infant suffers confusion between its natural desires and those of its parent. The result is frustration.

For such reasons, you should concentrate upon feeding and training programs for your child that will make him feel wanted and, at the same time, develop traits which will enable him to integrate easily with society. Demand breast feeding of your baby, if it is at all possible; late weaning; and still later induction of bowel training are the essential ingredients of such programs.

Over eighty per cent of all new mothers are capable of breast feeding, if they really want it. That is, the condition of their milk is nutritiously satisfying to the child, their nipples and breast tissue are structurally sound, and the act of breast feeding will not unduly tire them.

On the face of it, if you fall within this group, there is no reason why you should not breast feed your child. Besides gratifying your infant's wishes, as an emotionally mature woman you will derive a certain sensual pleasure from the baby's sucking. Thus joined with your child in an act of physical and emotional satisfaction, you will encourage a mutual feeling of love. Indeed, "breast-fed is the best fed" affords insurance for a healthy, happy infant.

We can go on to cite numerous additional advantages of breast feeding, such as the fact that breast milk is normally clean. And because there is no problem of storage, there is no possibility of deterioration. Nursing, too, is supposed to lower the incidence of breast cancer. But these are factors which any physician will discuss more fully with you before you decide whether or not you will breast feed your baby. The vital thing for you as a mother to remember is that tender, loving care can be imparted to the infant even by bottle feeding. Holding the baby close, allowing him to feel the warmth of the body, and real love are the factors that really count.

It would be unfair to suggest that hypnosis will automatically give you this insight and feeling. The chances are excellent, anyway, that you already have more than enough love to lavish upon your child. Still, hypnosis can do much more than relieve pain during labor and delivery. Its role in the post-partum period and beyond will be to help you keep your sights on the true goals of motherhood and, when you are exhausted physically and emotionally to the point where you "simply cannot take another step," to develop those reserves of untapped energy which we all possess.

In the following chapters we shall see how and why hypnosis can do all these things for you.

CHAPTER II

•

What Is Hypnosis?

HAVE YOU EVER had one of those days when practically everyone you meet stops and inquires: "Is something ailing you? You don't look well at all!"

You might have felt perfectly all right when you left home that morning, but by the third or fourth such inquiry your thoughts could be running something like this:

"I feel like a million dollars. I wonder why she thinks I look sick?

"There it is again. That's the second time today someone said I didn't look well. Maybe my make-up is on wrong.

"Say, I do look a little pale. I knew I shouldn't have gone out without a topcoat last night.

"There, I'm beginning to feel slightly warm. I've had this experience before. Once I get a fever, I have to stay in bed for a couple of days. Perhaps I should go home now and nurse the cold I'm getting."

We have all had such days. In almost less time than it takes to tell it, we have been transformed from pictures of radiant health to persons overly concerned with the slightest sign of illness. No matter how healthy we might be, suggestion can be so powerful an influence that we can be made to believe that we are less than well. It is equally well known that the effect of all this upon our physical being can be so great that we will actually develop many of the symptoms (aches and pains, etc.) of the disease we suspect we are catching—all because of suggestion or *our capacity to accept an idea uncritically.*

This fact is universally accepted by psychologists and physicians. An entirely new branch of medicine—psychosomatics—is based upon this capacity of the patient to "think" himself either sick or well. Parenthetically, we should add that such individuals are neither feigning nor imagining their symptoms, which can be as real as any of the well-known allergies and, in some cases, the common cold itself. In recent years the list of known psychosomatically-based diseases has been increased tremendously.

As students of hypnotism, though, we are concerned with how this phenomenon of "increased suggestibility" can be used to achieve healthy aims. We must, first of all, accept the definition that suggestion, in one manner or another, forms the basis for all hypnosis. Indeed, we shall be using the words interchangeably, because no one knows where suggestion ends and hypnosis begins. From this starting point, it is apparent that all of us have been literally "hypnotized" thousands of times without ever realizing it. The quiet ripples of a lake lapping against the side of our rowboat and lulling us into a relaxed state of mind, and the monotonous white line down the center of the highway inducing a feeling of drowsiness in us after many miles of constant driving—these are examples of hypnosis at work in our everyday lives.

Psychologists are fond of citing another instance of suggestion which can be helpful to most persons in one form or another. We can all walk a narrow board, say two feet wide, when it is placed on the ground, they tell us. Yet the same board, suspended twenty feet in the air, would represent a challenge impossible to meet unless we happened to be circus performers or we recognized that we had created this difficult situation for ourselves.

Why can we walk the narrow path along the ground and yet fail so dismally when the path is raised? The answer, of course, is suggestion. In the latter case, we "see" ourselves missing a step and being dashed helplessly onto the ground below. Therefore, we hesitate to perform a feat well within our physical capabilities. We are, in fact, victims of suggestions that we give ourselves, or "autosuggestions."

From all of the foregoing examples, we should be able to distinguish still another facet in our definition of hypnosis—a *narrowing of attention which effects our capacity to respond* to ideas and physical stimuli in the world around us. Certainly, this is not necessarily bad. We can, and do, use this limiting of sensory intake to a given idea or stimulus to good advantage in our more normal activities.

Notice the genuine music lover at a concert. He puts his head back, keeps both feet planted squarely on the ground, lets his arms fall naturally in his lap, and closes his eyes in order to hear better the blending of the instruments. Perhaps you have seen such individuals and even suspected that they were sound asleep. Exactly the opposite is true. The good music devotee knows that in this position he is more alert and better equipped to hear the concert than he would be if, eyes open, he was distracted by the waving of the baton or by the hat on the lady in front of him.

It might also be observed that the music itself produces a hypnotic or highly suggestive state in the listener. One of the first lessons we learn when we are very young is that the sound of a soft lullaby means "it is time to go to sleep." How many of us today can resist the urge at least to close our eyes when we hear those same melodies our mothers used to sing at our bedsides?

You must not assume from all of this that hypnosis is anything like being asleep. If anything, in a hypnotic state, an individual is wider awake than normally. Subjects hear and see everything that is going on about them. If, for example, some catastrophe, such as a fire, should occur while they are hypnotized, they will respond as rapidly as if they were in a normal state of awareness. And if they obviously concentrate upon the suggestions of the hypnotist, they do so because they have *confidence* in his ability to suggest ways of increasing their own happiness.

We are now at the crux of our definition of hypnosis, for without confidence there can be no suggestibility. Even when this confidence is present to begin with, it can be destroyed later on by a careless word or act on the part of the operator, at which point hypnosis abruptly ends. There is no substitute for confidence, and those persons who protest that they cannot be hypnotized are generally in reality saying: "I do not have confidence."

These, then, are the ingredients of hypnosis. Strung together, they read something like this: *Hypnosis is a favorable mental attitude or mind-set based on a blending of belief, faith, confidence, and expectancy, all fused through the imagination of the subject to produce increased susceptibility to suggestion.* Within the framework of this definition, your susceptibility to suggestion and/or hypnosis will begin the moment you first enter your doctor's office. Your confidence in his professional ability, and the expectancy that hypnosis will help you are the beginnings of a successful rapport.

But hypnosis does not demand blind faith from the subject. At first, you will, naturally, have a great many questions. You may even have some doubts concerning the effectiveness of suggestion. These are perfectly normal, for this is probably your first encounter with the professional use of hypnosis. Mature patients, though, come to their physicians with open minds. Their questions reflect an eagerness to learn. To help you overcome some of your own doubts, let us explore a few of the questions and answers most often heard in that first office visit.

CHILDBIRTH WITH HYPNOSIS

What are the real advantages to hypnosis?

Probably you are considering the use of hypnosis because you think it might be effective in relieving your pain and discomfort in childbirth. Actually, the control of painful sensations is one of the oldest uses of the art, but it is not the only reason people are hypnotized. The current popularity of the procedure, for instance, stems largely from the use of hypnosis as a form of psychotherapy in both World Wars. Thousands of fighting men who suffered crippling emotional disturbances in battle were returned to useful civilian lives via a combination of hypnosis and psychoanalysis called "hypnoanalysis."

This method of treatment is a means of circumventing lengthy and costly psychoanalysis through a phenomenon of hypnosis known as "age regression" or "memory recall." Under professional guidance, good subjects exhibit an almost limitless ability to recall events that were buried deep in their subconscious minds either because such events were too distasteful to remember or because they happened too long ago. Exposed to the scrutiny of a trained analyst, these memories can be a clue to abnormal behavior in certain cases of mental illness.

There is yet another facet to hypnosis which psychiatrists trained in hypnotic techniques find effective in their work, especially when the root of the difficulty lies in the patient's early formative years. This is the technique of "revivification," or the ability of a subject to relive a specific part of her life—no matter how far back the hypnotherapist may probe. A hypnotized person will, thus, perceive and behave exactly as she did at the time being recalled. Her speech, handwriting, and thought processes (including those things which frightened her) are so vividly relived that the subject lays bare those childhood experiences which crippled her adult personality.

Experiments in regression have produced startling as well as beneficial results. Instances of a subject's being regressed to the age of three or four years have been recorded. And in those instances where the subject has reportedly regressed to six or eight months of age, she will gurgle, coo, or cry as she did at that time in her life. However, this is usually due to role-playing, not regression. There is no scientific basis to the claim of some operators that they have succeeded in establishing regressions to the prebirth period. Finally, in all actual hypnotic regressions, the subject's return to her present age is speedily and easily affected.

There are, in addition to these, numerous advantages to hypnosis which are even less time-consuming and which are within the reach of most individuals. Subjects have successfully broken unwanted habits, cured themselves of insomnia or overeating, and just plain learned to live more relaxed lives with the techniques they discovered in formal hypnosis. At the heart of these "cures" is a phenomenon which we shall be mentioning frequently. It is "posthypnotic suggestion," or suggestions that might be given to a subject while she is hypnotized, but which do not become effective until a predetermined time after she is dehypnotized.

This technique is the basis for hypnotherapy in the treatment of many problems, but its use is not restricted to the physician. "After I am alerted, I will continue to feel pleasantly relaxed and unhurried no matter how many pressures I might have," a subject can tell herself with the same degree of effectiveness as if it were told her by her hypnotherapist.

Such suggestions are useful to your doctor, too. He might

venture the statement that the next time you visit his office he will be able to hypnotize you with less difficulty and in a shorter time. The example of rehypnotizing a subject by a gentle touch on her shoulder, mentioned in Chapter I, was an instance of this. And, of course, a subject's inability to feel pain even hours after formal hypnosis is terminated is still another beneficial use of posthypnotic suggestion.

While researchers have reported cases where a subject has performed a "suggested" act many years after she was hypnotized, such suggestions do tend to lose effectiveness with time. At most, we can count on their lasting only a few weeks. But because hypnotic training in childbirth seldom begins before the sixth month of pregnancy and is reinforced during periodic visits up to the time of delivery, we need not concern ourselves with this peculiarity of posthypnotic suggestion. Your hypnosis will remain a valuable ally at least throughout your pregnancy.

Are there any dangers or disadvantages to hypnosis?

The only real danger to hypnosis is that it is not dangerous enough. By this, we mean that the procedure is so safe and uncomplicated that it has inspired many amateurs and stage performers to try it. No matter how fumbling such attempts may be, they are not, in themselves, dangerous. Problems can, on the other hand, arise when these performers succeed in inducing hypnosis; these problems stem not from the hypnosis but from *what the hypnotists say and do while the subject is hypnotized.*

Very probably the majority of the commands will be harmless, if somewhat childish. We have all seen theatrical demonstrations of subjects barking as dogs, etc. Still, there is the possibility that these unprofessionals will unwittingly set off an emotional disturbance in a subject by suggesting an act which the individual may have been supressing for many years. If there is no skilled physician or psychiatrist present, the results can be damaging.

This undoubtedly accounts for the oft-heard false charge that hypnosis can change one's personality. Nothing can be more unfair to the professional use of hypnotism in medicine. It is true that physicians, through the use of words alone, can change one's outlook on life. A doctor performing a chest examination and listening to his patient's heart has only to say "um" and raise his eyebrows in a puzzled manner to make the individual suspect that there is something wrong with his heart.

In such instances, an otherwise healthy person might be made to display all of the symptoms of a hypochondriac. Yet it would not be just to blame the stethoscope or the fact that the doctor was listening to the heart for causing the patient's distorted point of view. So, too, it is not the hypnosis per se that might be responsible for untoward effects; rather, it is the suggestion that is given and the distortion of its meaning by a poorly-informed patient.

This is not to imply that hypnosis does not have some genuine disadvantages. First of all, it requires a great deal more time than some patients and physicians are willing to spend. The initial hypnotic induction might take anywhere from twenty minutes to an hour during the first office visit. As we have stated, though, this period can be reduced to a matter of mere seconds with posthypnotic suggestion in later visits.

Another disadvantage is that complete hypnotic anesthesia is simply not within the reach of all subjects. Results vary, of course, with the emotional make-up of the subject, the training of the physician, and the amount of time that both of them are willing to spend in teaching and learning deep hypnosis. Our experience tells us that better than ninety per cent of all obstetric patients can be hypnotized to some degree. These patients can often be relieved of most of the common discomforts of pregnancy, and the pains of labor can be mitigated. Although only less than one fourth of the women will require no chemical anesthesia at the time of delivery, the amount of anesthesia necessary in any case where the patient is conditioned in hypnosis is considerably below the average amount. And, in every instance of childbirth with hypnosis, there is less of an emotional "letdown" in the postnatal recovery period.

What do I have to do in order to become hypnotized?

To become a good hypnotic subject, you need, first of all, to keep an "open" mind. You should ignore the half-truths and gossip from well-meaning friends and relatives who might deride your decision to try hypnosis. When you arrive for your initial visit, you should listen and observe everything you can.

To insure the best possible chance of success for your hypnotic induction, you should have complete confidence in your physician. Certainly you should feel this way about all of your physician's recommendations, but, remembering our definition of the word, the feeling is essential for hypnosis. Finally, have faith in your ability to co-operate fully and to relax. In other words, arrive for your appointment expecting to be hypnotized—and you will be.

Once you set this "stage" for yourself, you will need only to listen to your physician's voice and to follow all the simple, elementary suggestions. For example, your doctor may tell you that your eyelids are getting heavy. It is imperative that you think, believe, and even feel your eyelids getting heavier at that time. If you cannot feel it, try imagining that you do. With just a little experience, you will be able to "pretend" almost anything. Later, as you permit yourself to feel most of the sensations that are suggested, this pretense will not be necessary.

Your hypnotherapist will have no way of knowing whether or not you are following his suggestions, but the degree to which you subjectively experience these suggestions will determine just how deeply you will go into the hypnotic state. Remember that hypnosis is due to increased susceptibility to suggestion and that before you can accept suggestions for such things as pain relief, you must first learn to accept the elementary suggestions of hypnosis.

How will I know when I am in a hypnotic state?

The first indication you will have that you are in a hypnotic state will be a wonderful sensation of relaxation coming over your entire body. If your feet are tired at the beginning of the session, this feeling will vanish as you turn your powers of concentration away from your feet and in whatever direction your doctor might suggest. It will be so easy to do this, and it will become increasingly difficult to let your thoughts wander.

In the beginning, your eyelids may feel weighted. They will seem to be so heavy that, at your doctor's suggestion, you will not be able to open them. Then, as your hypnosis deepens, you will be unable to open your eyes, but it will not be important to you whether you can or not. You will also notice a narrowing or riveting of your attention to the operator's voice. In other words, you will be listening very closely to his voice, and other sounds or distractions will fade away into the distance.

CHILDBIRTH WITH HYPNOSIS

The deeper you go into hypnosis, the more detached you will be from outside stimuli. When you are truly hypnotized, you will discover that you have a single-minded purpose that will not seem impossible to achieve. You will feel the desire welling up within you, and no task, within reason—physical or mental—provided that you truly want to accomplish it, will appear too difficult.

Can I be hypnotized against my will? Or can I be forced to do anything while I am hypnotized that I would not do in a normal state of awareness?

The answer to the former question is "most emphatically no!" And the answer to the latter, for all practical purposes, is the same. In thousands of cases of women we have hypnotized for professional purposes, we have not discovered one where the subject could be hypnotized against her will. As a matter of fact, it is somewhat misleading to state that we hypnotize anyone. The technique, as you must realize by now, is a step-by-step subjective procedure, with the subject permitting herself to go each step of the way. The hypnotherapist merely points out the direction. He does not, and cannot, push anyone into hypnosis. It is indeed a wise hypnotist who knows who is hypnotizing whom!

The mistaken notion that he can force someone into hypnosis probably originates with those stage performers who make much ado about the "Svengali" or "evil-eye" approach to hypnosis. They must present a picture of themselves as having deep, penetrating eyes and making passes with "magnetized" finger tips. To do otherwise would be to admit that hypnotism is a relatively easy practice which anyone can learn in a few hours.

The air of mystery is heightened, too, by creating the fear that subjects may be compelled to do evil things while hypnotized. We know of no such incidents, although there have been reports of experiments in which a hypnotized soldier in wartime attacked his commanding officer when told that the officer was really the enemy. Here, the perception and attitude of the subject were altered to produce the act. The circumstances surrounding these particular experiments could hardly be considered typical of an obstetrical situation, and the entire question becomes academic when we remind ourselves that physicians who use hypnosis are bound by the same code of ethics that they use in other facets of their practices.

What would happen to me if my doctor was forced to leave me while I was in a hypnotic state?

We have already observed that hypnotic rapport may be transferred from the physician to some other individual who can continue to lead the subject into deeper hypnosis. If, however, the hypnotist is compelled to leave abruptly, the subject would either lapse into deep sleep and then awaken spontaneously or come out of the hypnotic state immediately. Hypnosis is an interpersonal relationship between operator and subject. When either party disappears, the process of communication, naturally, no longer exists and the hypnotic rapport is terminated.

A far more common concern, however, is the case of an individual who remains in a deep hypnotic state despite the efforts of the hypnotist to bring him out of it. As scientists, we have investigated dozens of these situations over the past decade or so. In practically every instance, we discovered that the hypnotic state had been induced by an amateur or entertainer. Such an operator often embarrasses his subject by suggesting that he forget his name, behave like a child, or perform some ridiculous act while hypnotized.

The subject, anxious to appear a good sport and to please, performs against his true wishes. But later, when the hypnotist attempts to alert the subject, he meets resistance, because it is now the subject's turn to embarrass the operator.

In the medical approach to hypnosis, we eliminate the possibility of such a situation by permitting the patient the choices of whether or not she will go into a hypnotic state and at what pace she will proceed. Through instruction in autohypnosis, she has it well within her own power to alert herself whenever she so desires.

Is it possible to be just a "little bit" hypnotized?

Yes. It is not necessary to reach the deepest or "somnambulistic" state in order to benefit from hypnosis. The stages of hypnosis are not too well defined. Some subjects never seem to be able to get beyond the lightest stage, while others move on to the deeper stages without the doctor's being aware of it. The study of these stages is important to us only because the stages define the advantages that we might expect from each step along the way to the deepest hypnosis.

Nearly everyone can achieve the first light stage of hypnotizability. This is a condition of relaxation which requires only that the subject have an average intelligence. The imagination, rather than the will, is utilized. Note the word "imagination." Hypnotic susceptibility does not presuppose a weak will, a lowered mentality, or a strong mind over a weak mind. Quite the opposite is true. It is virtually impossible to hypnotize imbeciles or low-grade morons.

With just the ability to reach a state of light hypnosis, the average person can train himself to increase his capacity to respond to suggestions that are in full accord with his needs and wishes. He will also exhibit a pinpoint literalness that reflects a clarity of thinking comparatively rare in non-hypnotized individuals. To dramatize this point, we often request a subject to raise her *hand.* She responds by raising that portion of her body from her wrist to her finger tips. In better than nine cases out of ten, when a normally alert person is asked to perform this same act, he will raise an entire *arm.*

Unfortunately, even with the most skillful guidance, not all subjects will succeed in going "deeper" into hypnosis. The "cataleptic" or second stage is reserved for those who have the inclination, with the resultant ability, to enter deeper stages of hypnosis.

This second state is characterized by a marked muscular rigidity, which enables the subject to increase his physical efficiency by as much as twenty-five per cent. We observe this phenomenon in our patients who are asked to raise an arm upward as they feel themselves going deeper and deeper relaxed. When these subjects reach the cataleptic or medium state of hypnosis, it is difficult for one man or even two to bend their arms. Furthermore, subjects in catalepsy can keep their arms in an extended position for abnormally long periods of time without tiring.

Impressive! But for our purposes, the importance of the cataleptic state is that it is at this point that most subjects may begin to experience hypnotic anesthesia. The degree to which subjects will be able to withstand pain will generally increase as the hypnosis deepens. Almost anyone who can get beyond the first stage can be conditioned not to feel the pain of a needle pressed against his skin; but the ability to reduce the intensity of the labor contractions is reserved only for those capable of the still deeper states of hypnosis. In somnambulism, the deepest state of hypnosis, even a surgical incision can be withstood without pain.

What is the difference between hypnosis and the natural or "Read" method of childbirth?

To Dr. Grantly Dick Read, a British physician of world renown, both the medical profession and the women of the world owe a great debt of gratitude. With the publication of his *Natural Childbirth* in 1933, Dr. Read—who was himself stimulated by the pioneering efforts of such men as the late Dr. Joseph B. DeLee, founder of the world-famous Chicago Lying-In Hospital—brought into sharp focus a public awareness of the emotional reactions occurring during labor. He stated that the average woman in childbirth need have no more discomfort than she is willing to bear, and advocated less analgesia and anesthesia long before the current extensive research demonstrated the possibilities of fetal anoxia's being produced by excessive drugging.

Dr. DeLee, through his teachings and books, continued to be a leader among those who believed that labor is not the painful experience that generations of mothers have been led to believe. He did not deny the presence of pain during labor. Instead, he contended that suggestion in the form of the doctor's art effectively raised the patient's pain threshold, consequently reducing the need for harmful drugs. He stated that easily half the success of anesthesia in obstetrics was vocal! Dr. Read elaborated on Dr. DeLee's notions of making childbirth a satisfying experience by educating women in the psychological implications as well as the biological changes of childbirth. "It is impossible," he wrote, "to protect women from the fear of childbirth if they are ignorant of the truth. We do not fear facts, but doubts and uncertainties. Our most tremendous apprehensions arise from anxieties lest the worst may happen. Rumor is more terrifying than assault, ignorance more nerve-racking than knowledge, however bad reality may be."

We have no quarrel with these sentiments. In fact, we must wholeheartedly endorse the objectives of the Read Method as a step in the right direction. But, it does not go far enough! Hypnosis takes over where natural childbirth leaves off. Yet in both there is complete consciousness of the mother. However, in practice, when the Read Method is applied, pain-relieving drugs and chemicals are frequently used during labor and delivery and anesthetics are administered for the episiotomy and repair. So, we see, natural childbirth is not so natural as its advocates believe. Some degree of anesthesia is required by most patients using hypnosis; however, the anesthesia is needed in considerably lesser amounts.

One of the biggest differences between the Read Method and hypnosis is that the former is concerned primarily with the conscious fears and tensions of the pregnant woman while the latter, through subconscious mechanisms, *invokes the conviction* that fears and hidden anxieties will not lead to painful sensations. Hypnosis utilizes positive, constructive, and healthy conditioning to neutralize negative, destructive, and harmful conditioning to reverse faulty thinking patterns. It is a scientific "power of positive thinking" that works through the imaginative processes rather than the will.

Finally, the Read or "natural" method of childbirth involves a program of ritualistic procedures during the antenatal period. A course of some seven or more relaxing and breathing exercises for the pregnant woman to follow is outlined in Dr. Read's last book, *Childbirth Without Fear.* In advocating the practice of these exercises, the doctor explains: ". . . women who rarely exercise either their minds or their bodies bear their children with greater difficulty and more frequent interference than the peasant woman at the plow."

Again, those who advocate hypnosis for delivery are not at odds with this theory, although they doubt whether the exercises help the mother withstand pain. We doubt if the exercises described can condition a stenographer to the same degree, physically, as they can a farm worker. Surely this does not mean that a stenographer must always have more pain in childbirth. Without condemning such programs for the expectant mother, we prefer to fall back upon the words of Dr. Read himself: "The benefits derived from exercises are the same whether a woman is pregnant or not."

There are, of course, many of Dr. Read's principles, such as his contention that women deliver best in the squatting position, which are of more apparent merit. However, the value of his procedure lies less in the technique he employed and more in the confidence he inspired in his patients and the insight he gave them into childbirth. Although the doctor would probably be the first to deny it, we contend that the method he developed does use suggestion at different levels of awareness. Recognized or unrecognized, the success of all suggestive procedures is based upon the belief, faith, and confidence of the patient in her physician. The acceptance by her of him as an authoritarian figure, together with the expectation of pain relief, leads to the conviction that pain will be relieved. Nothing could be simpler.

The resultant favorable mental set or attitude leads to exaggerated suggestibility which may, in certain instances, spontaneously induce deep hypnosis, especially if the suggestions are repeated often enough.

Dr. Read was not conversant with hypnotic techniques. He believed that hypnosis was induced by the staring of eyes and the making of passes and was always accompanied by unconsciousness. He failed to recognize that individuals can enter into a hypnotic state without the necessity of a formalistic induction and that they often do not even know that they are in hypnosis. Dr. Read, in his naïveté, remarks: "Many of my patients appear as if in a trance near the end of the second stage." If this is not hypnosis, then what is it? Dr. Read's personal magnetism, charm, and prestige were the essential ingredients which relaxed patients approaching childbirth.

The reader can find everyday examples of this type of direct-prestige suggestion in exhibitions of successful entertainers, in salesmanship, and in spellbinding oratory. Physicians, too, consciously or unconscously use this form of suggestion in their practices and call it the "art of medicine." These doctors are only practicing what Voltaire preached when he said: "There is often more cure in the doctor's words than in the drugs he prescribes."

Perhaps for this reason Dr. Read's patients generally made excellent subjects for formal hypnosis. It has even been suggested that a combination of the Read Method with either light or deep hypnosis would result in still more comfortable labor. This is not difficult to imagine, just as long as the woman remains free to choose the path which best fits her personality.

CHAPTER III

•

Your First Steps Towards Relaxed Childbirth

NATURALLY, YOU WANT the very best care for yourself and your unborn child. Your obstetrician can provide this, first of all, if you consult him early in your pregnancy—generally two or three weeks after you first miss a menstrual period.

You need have no fears about this first office visit. For the most part, it will be a "get-acquainted" session between you and the doctor, who, along with his professional skills, has learned that this experience tends to be either needlessly confusing or embarrassing or downright frightening for most women. He will, therefore, do everything within his power to set you at ease the moment you step through the office doorway, and you should accept his sincere interest in your welfare in the same spirit as it is offered.

Before he begins to advise you how to have a healthy, happy pregnancy and delivery, your doctor will prepare a "case history" on you that will provide a basis for his recommendations. He will inquire as to your age, length of marriage, and number (if any) of previous pregnancies; how long it took to achieve the current pregnancy; and your normal weight. He will also ask a number of questions about your husband's health, as well as that of both your families, for as far back as you can remember. Of course, he will want your complete medical history. Are you diabetic? Do you have heart disease? Have you ever had measles? What operations have you undergone? In fact, you will probably have to reach way back to your childhood to come up with all the answers that your physician will require, but the rewards will be worth the small effort.

Very likely, too, your doctor will want to conduct certain tests to determine that you are, indeed, pregnant. There is no foolproof single test for very early pregnancy, but a number of these tests, coupled with the experience of your physician, will give both of you an answer upon which you may confidently rely. For one thing, an examination of your breasts, if you are pregnant, will reveal certain changes in the glandular tissue and pigmentation of the nipples. Then, too, changes in the tissues around the entrance of your vagina may indicate pregnancy to the professional eye of the physician, who may also feel the developing fetus in the uterus through the abdominal wall.

Other tests may be conducted in a laboratory, where a specimen of your urine will be injected into a small animal, such as a mouse, frog, or rabbit. Certain biological changes in that animal are near-positive proof that you are pregnant. Later in your pregnancy, around the end of the third month, your doctor may detect an outline of the fetus with X rays (the baby's first picture), and just a bit later he will be able to listen to its heartbeat.

Even while this history-taking and testing are going on, your doctor will inquire about your emotional attitudes towards life in general and your pregnancy in particular. These are every bit as important as your medical history, because, as you will soon discover for yourself, they have a very real bearing on the smooth course of your pregnancy, labor, and delivery. If your pregnancy is unplanned, or if either you or your husband is looking forward to the birth of your baby with dread, it is best to discuss this with your physician during that first office visit. He will discover the truth eventually, but he can save you months of needless suffering if he knows it at the start. On the other hand, if you and your husband are joyously anticipating the arrival of your child, your physician should know this, too. He is as anxious as you are not to complicate your life with un-necessary visits and instructions during the next eight or nine months. But, because no two pregnancies are ever exactly the same, your answers to his questions are the best guide he has.

Now you are ready for the physical examination. Of necessity, this will be a most personal one as far as you are concerned, but you should remember that your physician has examined literally thousands of women and that his attitude towards this phase of his relationship with you will be strictly impersonal.

You can expect this examination to be complete—from head to toe, including eyes, ears, nose, throat, heart, lungs, and thyroid gland. He will also do a urine analysis and give you a full blood test. At this time, your blood will be grouped into one of four main blood groups—A, B, AB, or O—in case a transfusion is necessary at delivery. Your blood will also be classified according to its minor blood type, either Rh positive or Rh negative. This Rh classification has been the butt of so much gossip and misinformation that it would take a volume just to set the record straight. Let us say only that no matter what the results of this typing, even if you are Rh negative and your husband is Rh positive, there is very little danger of your child's suffering because of the Rh factor—as your doctor can assure you. The Rh factor seldom involves the first-born, but combative measures do exist for those infants who are susceptible. Regarding the test itself, you will find it quite painless, since it involves only the drawing of blood by a needle and syringe from a vein of the arm.

During your first visit to his office, your obstetrician will also take your internal and external pelvic measurements —a presumptive indication, at this time, as to how difficult your delivery will be. He will, in addition, give you an internal examination to determine the size and position of your uterus. You might as well relax and co-operate during this examination, because it is only the first of many such examinations that you will have in subsequent months. They are necessary to gauge the amount of growth of the fetus and to check on the progress of your pregnancy.

When the examination is completed and your last question is asked and answered, you will probably be relieved to learn that you do not have to return for an office visit for an entire month. Most obstetricians see their patients at monthly intervals during the first five months of pregnancy. Later this interval is shortened to three weeks, and finally it becomes every two weeks or less in the eight-week period before the baby is born.

These subsequent visits are considerably shorter than the first. They are devoted mainly to urine analysis, weight measurement, and blood-pressure testing. During the last few months of your pregnancy, your doctor will begin listening to the fetal heartbeat to determine the position of your baby, and he will commence taking internal pelvic measurements to judge better how much assistance you might need in delivering.

Sometime around your sixth-month visit your physician may bring up the subject of what type of anesthesia you desire to have and how you want it. He may suggest some type of spinal block, gas inhalation, or local or novocain anesthesia. He may inquire whether or not you would like to experience one of the relaxation methods as natural childbirth or hypnosis. You should feel free to bring up this important matter yourself at any time—even during your very first visit—and discuss it frankly with your obstetrician. However, progress in the application of suggestive methods of childbirth as natural childbirth, psychoprophylactic relaxation, and hypnosis has been so swift and recent that the doctor knows, better than most patients, how really beneficial these procedures can be. Therefore, he is in an enviable position to discuss which type is applicable for you. Regarding hypnosis for childbirth, it should be optional or in accord with your wishes.

We discuss hypnosis with each patient early in her pregnancy. If she decides on it, this allows us plenty of time to educate her in all the aspects of hypnosis that will make the labor and delivery easier. It also permits sufficient time for the patient and doctor to get to know and trust each other better, thus establishing the healthy rapport so essential for effective hypnosis. Finally—and this is perhaps the most important reason of all—beginning the study of hypnosis early in pregnancy prepares the mind of the mother-to-be and leaves ample time for practicing the various techniques of inducing hypnosis until the mother-to-be finds the one which most comfortably fits her personality.

Hypnosis is suggested to almost all, or better than ninety-five per cent, of our patients. The very few exceptions are those women, at one end of the emotional scale, who are so motivated to begin with that, subconsciously, they seem to be relaxed, following the very principles of hypnosis that we are advocating. We do not consider hypnosis an either/or method, so we stress the fact that anesthesia will be available if needed. It is not our desire to build an impressive record of successes with hypnosis. And so, if it appears that we shall achieve the desired results without it, we simply let it go at that. Otherwise, we do not hesitate to use a combination of chemical anesthesia, such as novocain, with hypnosis.

The extreme neurotic patient, who obviously needs some sort of personal ego build-up, is usually rejected as a candidate for hypnotic childbirth. Into this neurotic group fall those obsessive, highly nervous individuals whose pregnancies are often an attempt to compensate for feelings of inferiority in their psychological make-up. Often these women will be the very ones who demand hypnosis, because they feel that it will enable them to overcome their deep-seated inadequacies or that it will at least give them a social status that they could not otherwise attain. While hypnosis can, and often does, help reduce pain in such cases, it is fraught with danger, because if the hypnosis is not entirely successful, the patient will feel that she has failed. This can further increase the emotional "letdown." This is not an indictment of the hypnosis; rather, it is another reason why the decision to use hypnosis should be left to qualified physicians.

Assuming that you are a reasonably adjusted person—and this does not mean that you are completely unafraid—and that you possess an average intelligence and imagination, your doctor may ask you to consider hypnosis. Remember that his suggestion is just that—a suggestion. He will never insist that you try it, and your refusal to go along with the idea will not cause you to "lose face" in the doctor's eyes. Habits and misinformation concerning hypnosis are, sometimes, so firmly imbedded in the patient's subconscious mind that it is impractical to try to overcome them in the brief time before childbirth. Furthermore, no obstetrician, no matter how well he is hypnotically-oriented himself, can hypnotize you if you are firmly against it.

Besides your regular physical examination—if you are interested—your office visit will be given over to a discussion of hypnosis, generally, and what it can do for you, specifically. Your doctor will explain that there are two main reasons why you should consider childbirth with hypnosis.

First, it will materially help you to make the remainder of your pregnancy free from discomfort. Second, during delivery, it will prove to be a relatively effective yet harmless form of anesthesia for both you and your child. These two chief advantages of hypnosis will be discussed, respectively, in Chapters VI and IX, "Hypnosis and Pain" and "Discomforts of Pregnancy." For the moment, let us eavesdrop on what might be a conversation between you and your physician during that crucial sixth-month visit.

"I don't know about hypnosis, doctor," you might say after he has explained the advantages and disadvantages of the procedure, as we have in Chapter II. "I don't think I've got the imagination to be a good subject. Besides, I think I'll feel a little foolish finding out."

These objections are extremely common. The very newness of the use of hypnosis in obstetrics makes some patients vaguely uneasy about trying it, and few individuals, other than artists, seem ready to credit themselves with even a normal imagination. Naturally, we cannot completely overlook the possibility that you truly would not make a good subject for hypnosis. About ten per cent of all of our patients simply cannot be hypnotized in the time available. But you can see that the chances are heavily in favor of your being at least hypnotizable. However, we do not have to guess. There is a simple way to find out for certain.

"We'll try a susceptibility test," your doctor will suggest.

"Susceptibility test?" you wonder, while visions of more needles in the arm or specimen-taking race through your head.

"It's quite simple," the doctor assures you. "I won't touch you at all. In fact, I'll just speak to you from this chair. The object of our little test will be to see just how good an imagination you do have and to introduce you to the very first stage of hypnosis. Just listen to the sound of my voice and try to imagine the things that I suggest.

"Don't worry, if you can't actually imagine some of the things we'll talk about, just pretend that you do. Later on it won't be necessary for you to pretend. You'll develop your imagination so that, very soon, you'll be able to see and feel anything you care to imagine.

"Now close your eyes and sit squarely in your chair," your doctor will say. "Put both feet flat on the floor in front of you and extend your arms straight out. . . . That's it. Palms down, please.

"I'd like you to imagine that I'm putting two lightweight, empty buckets on your hands. They're so light that you can hardly feel them. Even though your eyes are shut tight, you know that the buckets are there, because, in your imagination, you can see them . . . one on each hand. Listen only to the sound of my voice. . . . Put all other thoughts aside as you concentrate only on those buckets. You'll find that it is so easy to concentrate . . . so relaxing to think of just one thing.

"Imagine, if you will, that I am slowly pouring water from a pitcher into one of the buckets, either one that you choose. It's just a small amount of water, at first. I'm pouring slowly, and that bucket is getting just a trifle heavier.

"I'm pouring a little faster now. The bucket is about one quarter full, and you're beginning to feel the added weight on your hand. It's getting heavier and heavier. You can feel it pressing your hand downward. Not too fast, but very slowly . . . heavier and heavier.

"Keep your eyes closed and imagine how heavy that bucket is. It's more than half full now, and I'm still pouring slowly. It's getting harder and harder to keep your hand up. Now the heavy bucket on your hand is full of water.

Feel how heavy the weight is. It is pushing your hand down . . . down . . . and down.

"All right. Open your eyes."

Now was that little test not fun? Surely there was nothing mysterious or forbidding about it. Perhaps, too, you discovered that your imagination was pretty good after all. Did your hand with the "heavier" bucket end up a few inches or more below the other? Or did you resist the suggestions of heaviness so much that you finished the test with that hand actually higher than the other? It really does not matter which way your imagination took you. The important thing is that you exercised that imagination and, in so doing, learned how pleasant and relaxing it can be to sit back, close your eyes, and concentrate on one simple thought. If this was your first susceptibility test, you were probably amazed to discover, too, how powerful these simple thoughts can be. As a matter of fact, the reaction of most patients even to susceptibility tests is: "Where has this been all my life?"

The answer is: "Right in front of you all the time." We are all constantly responding to the suggestions of others: there's nothing new about it. For example, have you ever noticed what happens when just one person in a group yawns or when someone in a theater audience clears his throat, usually just before curtain time? Suddenly there is an epidemic of yawning or coughing—all because we are, every one of us, susceptible to a degree to suggestion.

Psychologists refer to this common stimulation of our muscles or glands by suggestion as an "ideomotor" response. But you do not have to yawn in a crowd, cough in a theater, or be a psychologist to see how this type of reaction works. When hungry, just think of a steak dinner smothered in onions or of some other favorite dish and note how your mouth begins to "water." Of course, your mouth would not "water" at the mere command to think of steak if you never in your life have tasted anything more flavorful than boiled meat and potatoes. Thus, we see that it is extremely difficult, if not impossible, to picture ourselves in a situation that we have never actually experienced. For this reason, your doctor will draw upon life's simplest experiences—those which are inherently present within you and in which you are most comfortable—to acquaint you with the remarkable powers of suggestion.

Naturally, each doctor/patient relationship is different, and so the particular susceptibility test that your doctor gives you may not necessarily be the same as the one mentioned above or even the same as the one that he gives other patients. He might, for example, omit a susceptibility test and get you started on your first steps towards relaxed childbirth simply by instructing you to sit comfortably with your eyes closed and your hands clasped tightly in front of you. Then he will suggest that if you *really* wish to go deeper relaxed, you will imagine that your hands are stuck tightly together. Surely, if you try long enough and hard enough, you will be able to get your hands apart. But if you wish to co-operate and believe the simple suggestions first, you will then be able to follow the later, more complicated suggestions, especially those conducive to your welfare—and that will be the beginning of deeper, more beneficial hypnotic susceptibility.

Although, by now, you should be convinced that you have absolutely nothing to fear from susceptibility tests, perhaps you are wondering about their real role in childbirth with hypnosis. As we have stated, one of the purposes of these simple little experiences is to give you some idea of how it feels to be hypnotized; but the tests do have other functions just as vital to your comfort. For one thing, they are designed to help you establish a full measure of confidence in your doctor/hypnotherapist, without which deeper hypnosis would be impossible. Another lesson to be learned from susceptibility tests—and if you learn nothing else, your progress will be insured if you learn this—is that *when the will and the imagination are in conflict, the imagination always wins.*

This is just another way of saying that no matter how much we *want* to do something, we cannot do it unless we also *imagine* that we *can* do it. We can, also, turn this lesson around and say that if we imagine that we *can* do something, we will *want* to do it. Both of these attitudes have an important relationship to hypnosis. They explain why, occasionally, we encounter the subject who sincerely wants to be hypnotized and who seems to follow every instruction, but who just cannot relax. The connection between the will and the imagination accounts, too, for the fact that the highly imaginative youngster generally makes a better subject than the older person more set in his thoughts and ways.

Well, how much imagination does it really take before hypnosis can be effective?

As you can observe from the foregoing examples of susceptibility tests—or the lightest stages of hypnosis—it does not take much. Let us take one final example of these tests to illustrate how far a little imagination can carry you. This one is called the "postural sway" test, and the object is to convince you, with nothing more than suggestion, that you are falling backward. There is absolutely no danger in your taking this test in your physician's office. He will use no props; nor will he even touch you. Yet in less than one minute, if you imagine it and follow his suggestions, you will temporarily lose your balance and fall back into his waiting arms.

To introduce this suggestion, your doctor will begin by standing a few feet behind you. "I want you to stand with your heels and toes together, your hands at your sides," he will say. "Look straight ahead. Be relaxed and just listen to me. In a few moments I will ask you to think of falling backward and, after a little while, you will find yourself falling backward. Do not be afraid. Just let yourself go. I will be right behind you to catch you. Here, let me show you how it will feel."

At this point, to demonstrate what is expected of you, the doctor may place his hands, gently but firmly, on your shoulders and pull you backward. It is only natural that you will take a step back to keep yourself from falling.

"You stepped back," the doctor will say. "That is exactly what you must not do. You did it because you were afraid that I might let you fall. But, you see, I was right there to catch you. We will try it again. This time, try to let yourself go completely relaxed. Don't be afraid. All right now, just relax. Hold your head up straight, close your eyes, and listen closely to what I say.

"Now I want you to think of falling backward. Imagine that you are falling backward, that a force is pulling you backward. In a few moments you will feel this force pulling you backward. It is there now, pulling you . . . pulling you . . . backward . . . backward. You are falling backward. You are falling. . . . You cannot help yourself. You are falling, falling. . . . Fall!"

In this example of the postural sway test, your belief that something would happen was heightened by the doctor's demonstrating what the fall would be like before any formal suggestion was made. And his confident statement, "You are falling. . . . Fall," was calculated to produce just such an air of expectancy in you.

Do you feel now that you would like to go deeper into this wonderful, exciting subject of hypnosis? If, at this, the conclusion of your introduction to hypnosis, your head is spinning with thoughts of the new world which has been opened to you, do not worry. It is a perfectly normal reaction from patients who have been introduced to the facts about hypnosis for the first time. The important thing to remember is that it is virtually impossible not to enter some degree of hypnotic relaxation. Your physician will work as long and patiently with you as he thinks is necessary to set you at ease in this new atmosphere. Also, you need not analyze what he will say during the initial induction. Indeed, it will be better if you do not. By not analyzing what *will* be said, you will be better able to direct your awareness towards what *is* said.

From here on in, both your progress with training in hypnosis and your pregnancy should be smooth and rapid. Soon your baby's movements will be quite discernible. Very likely you will begin to feel the baby kicking you and will even observe it moving against your abdominal wall. And while your doctor continues to check on the health of you and your child, he will gradually introduce you to the phenomena of still deeper hypnosis. There is no denying that the relief of pain and the other advantages of hypnosis can be achieved only through hard work on your part; and the best results are usually obtained in the deeper stages of relaxation. After you read the next chapter, you will discover for yourself how it is possible to go from one relaxing state to the next. But, for the present, you need only remember to keep each office appointment faithfully and to go to as many training classes as possible so that you can learn more about hypnorelaxation.

There is one thing more that your physician will recommend to make your introduction to hypnosis gentle and effective in the final months of your pregnancy. It is that you supplement visits to his office by attending the above-mentioned group training classes in hypnosis. These are usually twice-monthly sessions of about two hours each conducted by the doctor in either his office or the hospital. There you will meet some dozen or more other women who are planning childbirth with hypnosis. Almost all of them, like yourself, will have had no previous experience with hypnosis, so you need not be afraid or ashamed to ask whatever questions come to mind during these group get-togethers. It would be a good idea, too, to bring your husband to these classes. He will find them a rewarding experience, because the benefits of hypnosis go far beyond comfortable childbirth. Then, too, with this knowledge he will be more understanding of your practice sessions at home. Most important of all, you will enjoy opening this trunkful of knowledge together.

Your first group lesson will be devoted mainly to a résumé by the doctor of what hypnosis is, what it is not, and what you can accomplish with it during labor and delivery. Its limitations and the popular misconceptions about it will be discussed in detail. All of the classes will also feature a demonstration, by four to six patients who are good hypnotic subjects, of how easily hypnosis can be induced by just a few words from the doctor. Additionally, most of the patients will demonstrate self-hypnosis and self-dehypnotization. Volunteers for this part of the meeting are usually housewives who have had no previous experience with hypnosis but who, in the office visits, have displayed an ability to enter readily into various stages of hypnosis. Perhaps, after you have gained a measure of self-confidence, you will find yourself volunteering for a role in this part of the evening in order to help some other woman feel more comfortable. The volunteer subjects not only permit themselves to be hypnotized but also demonstrate "glove anesthesia" (self-induced anesthesia of the palm), showing how, with it, they can make themselves virtually insensible to pain anywhere in the body.

Your doctor—or his associate, who might be conducting the class—will ask the entire audience to participate in group hypnosis. You should, if you are not acting as a volunteer, take part in these proceedings. Here, hypnosis is designed to familiarize you with the techniques you will later on encounter. As we mentioned earlier, it matters very little if you fail to react to all suggestions at this time. A little practice and lots of patience will change that; but in order to know what to expect of yourself, you ought to participate in these sessions at every opportunity.

Another vital portion of the group training class will be given over to those who have already experienced childbirth with hypnosis, either with or without drug sedation and chemical anesthesia. These women will recite details of how they felt during their pregnancy and delivery and will be very happy to answer any questions from the audience about their experiences with hypnoanesthesia. The unrehearsed story of the average woman will be straightforward and in language that you can readily understand. The following account, transcribed at one of these group sessions, is fairly typical of what you can expect to hear.

"I arrived at the hospital at about 7:15," this hypnosis-experienced woman told the others. "The contractions were coming about two or three minutes apart. I had some difficulty relaxing in the car on the way over, because I was unable to lie down. However, I was not really uncomfortable until the time came to expel the enema. I thought, at that time, that I was in the transition between the first and second stages of labor, because I was no longer able to relax during the contractions, but, instead, I felt the irresistible urge to push that one feels during the second stage.

"It is hard to distinguish this sensation from the very similar feeling connected with expelling the enema. There was no one immediately present to question about how far along I was, and, as a result, I was distressed for fear my baby would be born along with the enema. But I reasoned that, if the nurse who had just given me the enema had suspected I was so near delivery, she never would have left me alone. Nevertheless, I was very uncomfortable during those few minutes, both physically and mentally. I did not have pain, though, in the sense that I had pain while delivering my first child [without the benefit of hypnosis].

"Back on the bed in the labor room, I was immediately more comfortable. I tried relaxing again during contractions, thinking that perhaps the urge had been due to the enema, but I could not relax well. About this time, my doctor came in and examined me. He asked if I wished to have any assistance. I decided that I would like help in relaxing. He then asked me to close my eyes at a count of three, breathe deeply, start counting slowly, and relax. This deepened my feeling of relaxation at once and induced a tingling feeling of numbness in the tips of my fingers, making them feel so stiff that I could not bend them.

"Still, I was completely conscious and retained a sense of being in control of myself. In fact, I felt that if I had strongly wished to bend my fingers I could have done so.

CHILDBIRTH WITH HYPNOSIS

My doctor left the labor room, and my husband came in. I was perfectly conscious of his presence and glad that he was there holding my hand, but I felt no desire to speak with him or with anyone else except insofar as they could be of help to me in doing my job. The only real thought I had was to have a normal, healthy baby.

"My contractions were coming so fast that there was almost no space between them. I heard my husband tell the doctor that they were about one minute apart. Presently, without thinking whether or not I had reached the end of the first stage, I found myself bearing down. This was not a planned action. I simply found myself doing it. My breathing was extremely heavy, and I heard myself making the strange grunting noise with each push that had frightened me when I was delivering my first baby. After a few of these, I felt the bag of waters break. My doctor examined me. I was transferred to a cart and taken to the delivery room. I remember feeling very annoyed at the interruption in my work caused by the transfer to and from the cart.

"On the delivery table, I had no interest in anything but the one job of pushing. Much as I wanted the baby, I don't believe I was thinking any further ahead at that stage than just pushing. I was certainly not comfortable, but I had no pain.

"It was simply like the feeling one might have before having the biggest bowel movement imaginable. I was very calm. My doctor kept telling me what was happening, and how I was progressing, so that I could define every sensation. *For the first time in my history of childbirth, I felt that my presence as an emotional human being as well as a reproductive system was being recognized.*

"I remember that my doctor asked me if I wanted to see my baby born, and I replied that I did. Only later did I discover that, in the excitement of feeling the baby born, I forgot to open my eyes so that I might see it as well. There was a tremendous feeling of tension, just before the head was born.

"Then, I felt the body slither out without any further effort. I was greatly relieved and satisfied. I opened my eyes and saw the doctor holding my little girl all messy and wriggly. She was still attached to me by her cord. I felt such a surge of affection and pity that I surprised myself. It was then that I realized what a real crime it is to deprive a woman of consciousness at the birth of her child.

"There is a vital emotional need to experience fully the final and most dramatic act in the creation of a life," this woman continued. "When the continuity of creation is broken, the process does not seem complete: the end product—the child—seems somewhat remote. There is not the easy transition from thinking of the child as a concept, or a physical part of oneself, to recognizing it as a new human being complete unto itself.

"The transition is, at best, a tremendously complicated one—it is always difficult to part with a bit of oneself. Yet, since the parting is inevitable, how much better to experience it fully at the moment of its physical happening, so that it is faced at once and recognized, than to drag the need for it through one's subconscious long after the child is born.

"It seems to me a curious scientific lag," she concluded, "that doctors and nurses still sometimes act as though they believed in the old theory that mind and body are separate, and their concern is exclusively with the body. This is especially surprising when it concerns maternity cases, because the whole process of conception, prenatal activity and development, and the birth itself are so highly charged with emotion."

CHAPTER IV

•

"Deeper Relaxed"

ASIDE FROM YOUR physical examinations, the last office visits during your pregnancy, provided that you are not attending the group classes, will be given over to training you in the techniques of developing "glove anesthesia" and deeper, and still deeper, relaxation—or hypnosis. Actually, this procedure will not be much different from the susceptibility tests you took earlier. However, instead of suggesting that you feel some imaginary weight or that your hands are stuck tightly together, your physician will suggest that you gradually relax every muscle in your body. Naturally, you will not be expected to do this all at once. Certain muscles, such as those in your eyelids, toes, and fingers, are easier to relax than others. It might take some practice before you can relax the muscles around your thighs, arms, and abdomen and reach the depth of hypnosis necessary for anesthesia. In fact, if you cannot achieve this degree of relaxation by the sixth visit or so after you begin learning about hypnosis, your physician will probably suggest that you concentrate only upon relieving some of the discomforts of pregnancy with hypnosis and leave the relief of pain to more conventional methods.

If this should happen to you, do not consider your experience with hypnosis a failure. Many women who cannot reach anything but the lightest stage of relaxation throughout their pregnancies still find that it stands them in good stead during labor and delivery. After all, twenty to thirty per cent of hypnosis is still better than none at all. At most, such patients require only mild doses of chemical anesthesia. Furthermore, progress through the practice of even light hypnosis is so gradual, but so sure, that highly-motivated patients often amaze themselves by "forgetting" all about anesthesia except, perhaps, for the episiotomy and repair, if that procedure is necessary.

It is certainly best that you arrive for your remaining office visits dressed as comfortably as possible. Your doctor will advise what type of clothing you should be wearing now for your physical as well as for your emotional comfort. Generally, aside from other maternity outerwear, the prescribed clothing will include shoes with low, flat rubber heels; a snug-fitting, but not too tight, maternity brassière; a comfortable, well-fitting maternity girdle; and suspensory garters rather than the circular variety. These things will contribute to your over-all feeling of well-being and will have a very real function in maintaining your physical health. If, in addition, you look forward to having your baby with a feeling of joy and happiness instead of one of dread and anticipation between visits, your labor and delivery will be that much more effective.

Despite what you may have heard, your physician will not use drugs to facilitate hypnosis; nor will anything other than suggestion be needed to hypnotize you. Actually, you are the one who achieves the hypnosis, primarily because you want it. It is true that certain chemicals, such as sodium amytal or pentothal, if given in proper doses, may increase the susceptibility of an individual to suggestion: but this, in itself, is dangerous during pregnancy. Following the induction of hypnosis, a rapport between the physician and his patient is established. This bond of understanding and confidence cannot be forged by any chemical known to medicine today. Therefore, there is no substitute for words and the strength of the interpersonal relationship. As any woman who has had a baby will attest, this relationship has a highly sedative effect on every anxious mother-to-be in labor. Even her doctor's presence is conducive to relaxation.

Your doctor will, more than likely, adhere to the purely permissive approach to hypnosis and, to relax you further, will use a method of induction that is compatible with your desires. In this technique you are told that you are going to be relaxed and that if you concentrate on his suggestions and accept them, you will be able to relax when "the chips are down" during labor. The doctor will never deceive you; nor will he expect you to deceive yourself. In short, you will be expecting and looking forward to the induction of hypnosis and auto- or self-hypnosis.

One of the first things your doctor might do, after he has allayed your fears that you could not be hypnotized, is to direct your attention to how you breathe. That may seem strange, considering that breathing is something you have practiced for a lifetime. But the *way* you breathe can indicate how you feel even though you may not say a word. If you are tense and anxious, your breathing will be more shallow and rapid than it is when you are relaxed and unafraid. This reaction is involuntary. You can no more control it than you can hold your breath indefinitely. Furthermore, it is impossible to take deep, regular breaths without noticing some feeling of relaxation coming over you almost from the very first exhalation. Despite the fact that most persons have learned this lesson at one time or another, they seldom practice it, because breathing is so habitual that few of us stop to think about it.

You will begin your session, then, by inhaling deeply and exhaling slowly several times. Next, your doctor will invite you to seat yourself comfortably in a chair, with both feet squarely on the floor and your hands resting naturally in your lap. "You will please look up at a spot on the ceiling directly over your forehead," he may say. "Don't move your head, just your eyes. Let them roll way back . . . the farther the better . . . until they fasten on that spot on the ceiling.

"Keep staring at that spot, and, as you keep looking, you will soon notice that your lids will get heavy, very heavy. . . . And, as your lids get heavier and heavier, you will wish to close your eyes.

"Just keep looking at that spot. . . . Now, if you really wish to go into a deep state of relaxation, it is so easy to do, because all you have to do is imagine . . . think . . . and feel that your eyes are getting very, very heavy. As a matter of fact, at the count of three, if you really wish to relax deeper and deeper, you will let your eyes close. You will notice that your eyes will be locked tighter and tighter together.

"One: your eyes are getting heavier and heavier. . . . Two: your lids are getting heavier and heavier, and very, very tired. As your lids get heavier and heavier, it is going to feel so good to close your eyes. Then, after your eyes are closed tight, you will go deeper and still deeper relaxed. Your eyes are closing. One . . . two . . . three. Shut your eyes tight, tighter, and tighter. Let your eyeballs roll up into the back of your head, as if you were looking at your hair. And, as your eyeballs roll upward, you will notice that your lids are sticking together tighter and tighter.

"If you wish to go deeper, just tell yourself that your lids are locked tight, and then tighter. Say, 'I cannot open them.' All right. . . . Now keep your eyes closed and breathe slowly and naturally. With every breath you take, you are getting more and more relaxed. And, if you really wish to, you may go even deeper relaxed . . . with each and every breath. It is so easy to do. Simply listen to my voice."

Can you follow these simple instructions? If so, you will make a very good subject for hypnosis because, while your physician may vary the procedure somewhat with different patter, this is all it takes for you to enter the first stage of formal hypnosis. Of course, there are any number of other excellent methods that the skilled doctor can use to heighten your susceptibility to suggestion and to induce relaxation. Almost all of these, though, begin with the monotonous repetition of some simple suggestions. Your physician may ask you to count backwards slowly from one hundred or to focus your eyes on a real spot or a pinpoint of light rather than on an imaginary spot. Some doctors prefer working with more elaborate setups, such as the beat-beat-beat of a metronome or the movements of a whirling disc. However, in each instance, the object is the same—to narrow your attention to the suggestions of your physician and to create an atmosphere of expectancy and acceptance of what he has to say. It is only natural that if "a pipeline of communication" is established with you and there is "no static on the circuits," the message you receive will be ungarbled.

If you have co-operated so far and allowed yourself to enter this initial or light stage of hypnosis, you will notice an increased receptivity taking place in your feelings and attitudes. In the first place, you hear better with your eyes closed, and you will find it easier to act on the suggestions of your doctor. And there is really nothing very mysterious about any of this. The difficulty in opening your eyes, for example, is due to the placement and length of the muscles around the eyes rather than to any "power" of the doctor. Try it, right now, and see. The purpose of incorporating this little experiment in the hypnosis procedure is to direct your attention to a specific task and to make relaxation from the strain of trying just that much more inviting.

Once you cease trying to open your eyes and permit yourself to relax, you will notice other unusual, but pleasant, sensations taking hold of you. If your doctor tells you that one of your arms is getting lighter than the other and that it is so light that it is beginning to float upward, you will feel it becoming lighter without any conscious thought or effort on your part. It will seem almost as if you are standing outside of yourself observing such effortless movements. For perhaps the first time in your life, you will set your own pace for thinking as well as for moving about. There will be no thought of rushing the hypnosis or of worrying about any of the so-called "normal" cares of the day. It will seem to you that you are on a happy vacation. In this sense, hypnosis is truly an opportunity to step temporarily outside of yourself; but remember that you may pick up the hectic "normal" life whenever you wish.

While you will, certainly, have all of the freedom of choice that we just mentioned, you will discover that it is much more satisfying to follow the directions of your doctor. He will never ask you to do or feel anything which you do not want to do or feel. Therefore, you will have no reason to resist his suggestions. Instead, you will direct your thoughts to whatever part of your body he may suggest. For example, if he asks you to concentrate on your finger tips, you will do just that. When you do, you will discover how much control you have over the sensations at your finger tips. You can make the tips feel warm, cold, or numb by just thinking about it. In other words, you are now learning how to control your body functions instead of letting them control you! A bit later on, we shall see how this last phenomenon is useful in inducing hypnoanesthesia.

CHILDBIRTH WITH HYPNOSIS

Hypnosis is a pleasant experience. To be truly effective, it cannot be otherwise. Yet, by now, you are probably beginning to wonder how you can return to the rushed, anxious, but more natural state you were in before all this began. Never fear that your physician will leave you permanently hypnotized. That is impossible. Most likely, if he left you in a relaxed state, you would simply either bring yourself out of it or decide to fall into a deep, natural sleep and "awaken" normally. In any case, your experience with hypnosis would end with no ill effects. However, reputable physicians do not leave their patients hypnotized. Actually, to do so is impossible: since you were the one who let yourself enter into this relaxed state, you can bring yourself out of it at any time—even when you are in the deepest of hypnotic states. When the session is ended, you will find that your doctor has an effective routine for bringing you back to the nonhypnotic state.

"And now I'm going to alert you," he will say, "by calling off four letters of the alphabet—A, B, C, and D. You will be able to open your eyes slowly. In fact, you will be able to open your eyes completely when I say the letter D.

"You will feel fine—relaxed and completely refreshed. You will look forward to going still deeper and more relaxed the next time. You will feel very happy and thoroughly relaxed . . . as if you'd slept for several hours.

"That's right; open your eyes slowly now, feeling very relaxed and happy . . . as if you'd had a long, comfortable sleep. Listen to me call off those letters to you. . . . A . . . B . . . C . . . slowly . . . now D. . . . Open your eyes —feeling wonderful. You will look forward to having your baby with a feeling of joy and happiness instead of dread and anticipation. Remember, also, at no time were you asleep, unconscious, or in a so-called 'trance.' Rather, you heard everything I suggested—everything. That is why we use hypnosis—to get you to concentrate on everything I say; and if you pay attention to what I say, you will follow all suggestions that you wish to. Again, may I emphasize that you were not asleep. [Note that the phrase *wake up* is never used, as the subject is never asleep but is in a state of hyperalertness. The terms *awake* and *asleep* only confuse the picture.] Sleep and hypnosis are not the same. If you were asleep, obviously you wouldn't be able to hear my suggestions or even act on your own."

And so, because you want to, you will safely and speedily return to a normal state of awareness of your surroundings. You will open your eyes and be aware of where you are and what you are doing there. The feeling will be very similar to that of arising from a deep sleep; it will be the same sense of well-being, peace, and contentment. In the case of sleep, this feeling usually lasts just long enough for you to put your feet on the bedroom floor and make your first decision of the day. Then a million and one minor distractions crowd your thoughts, so that you find it difficult to concentrate on a major project. With hypnosis, though, the healthier, relaxed outlook may last much longer because, as you will discover before you have finished the last chapter of this book, you have it within your power to keep right on reinforcing these attitudes of contentment.

Whether or not you will remember what was said to you or what happened while you were hypnotized depends upon the suggestions of your physician. Many doctors tell patients who are capable of entering deep hypnosis or somnambulism that, after being alerted, they will recall nothing that transpired during hypnosis. This is known as posthypnotic amnesia. It can occur in about twenty per cent of all hypnotic inductions. You have the final say as to whether or not you wish to have a partial or total loss of memory for any of the practice sessions or for any portion of the labor/delivery.

Later, when you are using hypnosis to see you comfortably through childbirth, your physician will suggest that you will forget any part of your labor. For practical purposes, you will not have experienced any painful sensations. Yet, if you wish to do so later, you can recall everything else about your labor and delivery. You will always be free to remember or forget whatever you wish—this is called "selective amnesia." Some women choose to "put themselves out" entirely. "Where am I? How did I get here?" one of our patients asked immediately after she gave birth to a healthy nine-pound boy with no other anesthesia than hypnosis. "My mind was a complete blank," she said. "And if you should ask me to write about this experience, I would hand you a blank piece of paper." This is total amnesia.

With each visit to your doctor's office, you will need less and less time to become completely relaxed. When you are finally ready to go to the hospital to have your baby, it will take no more than a few seconds to induce deep hypnosis.

"All this is very well, if my hypnosis follows the one-two-three pattern outlined here," you may say. "But what happens if I'm in that group, small though it may be, who just cannot be hypnotized easily?"

We have already stated that your doctor will continue trying, for at least six visits, before he assumes that you cannot be hypnotized. It would be grossly unfair if, during these attempts, you were to compare the doctor unfavorably with some stage performer who apparently hypnotizes a greater percentage of his subjects. Remember that the performer can hand-pick his good subjects and thus bypass the resistant subject in favor of one who will make him look good. On the other hand, the doctor must continue to work with every patient who wants to be helped with hypnosis, whether she is apparently susceptible or not. If, after everything you have learned about hypnosis, you still fall in this latter group, your doctor may try a technique of hypnosis known as the levitation method of induction. This procedure will require even less co-operation on your part than the method described above, and it will enable you to begin the induction with your eyes open.

Your doctor may ask you to sit comfortably in a chair with the palms of your hands on your thighs. He will tell you to look at your hands and to keep staring at them. Then he will ask you to press down tightly with the palms on your thighs, as though you are pushing your feet into the floor.

"Press tighter and tighter," he will say. "As you keep pressing tighter and tighter, you will notice that one of your fingers will get lighter than all the rest. It may be the little finger on the left hand or the middle finger on the right hand. Perhaps it is the right ring finger or the index finger on the left hand. It doesn't really matter which, because, if you really wish to go into a deep, deep state of relaxation, *you will choose* one of the fingers on either hand to get lighter and lighter. . . . There, one of your fingers is beginning to twitch."

At this point, depending upon how well you are concentrating on what the doctor is saying, you may experience any one of a number of reactions. Because the pressure of pushing downward produces an uneven flow of blood to your finger tips, you may actually feel one finger getting lighter than all the rest. Then again, even though you do not really sense it, you may imagine that you feel the lightness, or you may ignore the help that you are getting and persist in your resistance by telling yourself that nothing is happening. It cannot be overemphasized that the choice is yours, not the doctor's.

Actually, "imagining" is one of the better responses. Just as the good stage actor must become so emotionally involved in the role he is playing that he seems to "live" the part, you must convince yourself that certain phenomena are occurring. Do not worry because you feel that you might not be good at this game of pretense. In the hand levitation method of induction, the things that you will have to imagine are especially simple.

"You have a desire to raise this finger up, up, and up," your doctor might suggest. "It is getting lighter and lighter than all the rest. You can take your time in making this finger lighter. It may require one second, one minute, or several minutes. But after your finger has got lighter, you will begin to feel that same sensation in all the fingers on that hand."

Here is where we begin to leave pretense behind. You are on your way towards being hypnotized if you can "feel" the lightness that your physician is suggesting. In other words, the first necessity of hypnosis—belief—commences to take hold when you realize that what your doctor is saying is true. Concentrate and feel these sensations. It will be impossible to reach this stage without following his suggestions, and it is this concentration on pleasant thoughts that will push any fear or anxiety that you may have farther and farther into the background.

"And, as you are pressing down with all the fingers of your hand," you will hear your physician say, "you note, too, that there is an increased sensitivity of the fingers. You can feel the texture of the clothing you are wearing, and you are aware, perhaps, of the warmth of your body through the cloth. As you continue to press down and develop this increased sensitivity, you notice that the finger which is lighter than all the rest is beginning to rise. It is so pleasant to let it get lighter and lighter. It is so relaxing. Now if you want to go still deeper and deeper relaxed, you will close your eyes and let all of the fingers on that hand get so light that they will want to raise off the thigh. Soon the entire hand will get very, very light and begin to rise. And, as your hand goes slowly upward, you will become deeper and deeper relaxed. Your arm is *lifting, lifting, lifting,* higher and higher."

If your arm continues to lift up toward your face, you need have no doubts about either your ability to be hypnotized or the fact that other suggestions that you will receive while in hypnosis will make the remainder of your pregnancy more comfortable and the birth of your child more rewarding. No matter which technique works best for you, the immediate result will be a nice sense of relaxation and an even greater confidence in your own ability to relax or to terminate even the deepest state of relaxation. In either case, too, the "alerting" procedure will be basically the same as the one mentioned earlier. There is no relationship between the difficulty you may find in accepting hypnosis and the return to a normal state of awareness.

At this stage in your training, both you and your physician will want to take stock of what you have accomplished so far. In the first place, you will discover that, now, you can go completely relaxed within seconds after you enter your physician's office. The method of induction by the doctor will be simple, direct suggestion, or something like this: "All right, now. Just close your eyes and start counting slowly backward from ten. By the time you reach seven, your eyelids will get very, very heavy. At the count of five, you will close your eyes and begin to go deeper and deeper relaxed. When you reach three, you will be completely relaxed." To make it easier for you to respond to this simple approach, at sometime before the end of each visit the doctor will suggest that your next session with hypnosis will be easier and swifter. This is just one of the uses of the phenomenon of posthypnotic suggestion that we touched upon in Chapter II.

To your physician, the hypnosis has an importance all its own. For one thing, in the relaxed state, when your "guard is down," he will learn more about your fears, anxieties, and tensions than he would in hours of questioning you under "normal" distracting circumstances. Gradually, then, he will adapt his hypnotic technique to your likes and dislikes. The examples of induction which we have been discussing are just that—examples. For reasons known only to you and your subconscious mind, you may be uncomfortable imagining some of the things we have suggested. Your physician will quickly detect this in the earliest visits and will shift to suggestions more compatible with the needs of your personality. Hypnosis is not personality analysis. While it is interesting to speculate upon *why* certain suggestions work well with some people and not so well with others, your doctor is more concerned with what your problems are and how you react or respond to them.

Another important fact about the initial stage of hypnosis is that it enables the subject to pass from the light into still deeper stages of relaxation. Many of the more beneficial phenomena of hypnosis, such as the relief of pain, usually can be accomplished only when the subject is in these deeper stages. And, after a good beginning, you need have no fear of deeper hypnosis, which is only, actually, a continuation of the relaxation and concentration process. As you permit yourself to go deeper and still deeper, the suggestions of your doctor sink in and are indelibly imprinted in your brain. You will have no difficulty concentrating, because outside noises recede farther into the background and, most important of all, you sense an upsurge in your ability to master sensations within your own body. After all, if you imagined heaviness and lightness, it will be easy for you to accept anesthesia without question through such suggestions as, "You will feel no pain."

Just how deep you will have to go and how long it will take for you to reach the depth of relaxation necessary are strictly up to you. We have known excellent subjects who passed from the lightest to the deepest stages of hypnosis in just one visit; but they are the exceptions. More consistently, we find that once hypnotic rapport is established, seventy-five per cent of our patients achieve a depth of hypnosis suitable for inducing some degree of anesthesia sometime before the tenth office visit. The stage that these patients reach is called the "cataleptic" stage of hypnosis because, as we shall presently discuss further, we know that it is one in which we can induce a catalepsy, or muscular rigidity. The increased stiffness is used as a test to let you and your doctor know that a medium stage of hypnosis has been attained.

There are still deeper stages of hypnosis, of course. These range all the way to the deepest, or "somnambulistic," stage, and each is marked by certain phenomena which generally are not produced in any preceding stage. But, aside from knowing that they exist, you need not concern yourself much with these various degrees of hypnosis. You will hardly ever realize when you pass from one stage to the next. Your doctor, though, knows that the degree to which you follow his suggestions increases your susceptibility and, as a result, increases the depth of your hypnosis. For this reason, his interest in deeper relaxation has been the object of considerable research. One of the first attempts to define how deeply hypnotized a subject must be in order for a specific suggestion to be effective was reported in the *Journal of Abnormal and Social Psychology* in 1931 by doctors L. W. Davis and R. W. Husband. The gist of their "Hypnotic Susceptibility Scoring System" is reported below for the benefit of those patients who might be asking themselves: "Where do we go from here?"

HYPNOTIC SUSCEPTIBILITY SCORING SYSTEM

Hypnotic Depth	Objective Symptoms
Light or "Hypnoidal" state	Relaxation Fluttering of eyelids Closing of eyes Complete physical relaxation
"Cataleptic" state	Catalepsy of eyelids Limb catalepsies Body catalepsy *Anesthesia*
Medium hypnosis	Partial amnesia Posthypnotic anesthesia Desirable personality changes Simple posthypnotic suggestions Delusions of heat, etc.

Hypnotic Depth	"Deeper Relaxed" Objective Symptoms
Deep or "Somnambulistic" state	Ability to open eyes without affecting hypnosis More complex posthypnotic suggestions Ability not to "hear" distracting sounds Ability not to "see" distracting sights Deepest relaxation

It is quite easy to pass from the lighter stages of hypnosis to the more rewarding depths of relaxation. When your physician decides that you are ready for, let us say the cataleptic stage, he will induce light hypnosis and then direct you to concentrate only upon his suggestions. "Nothing else seems to matter," he will say. "And nothing will disturb you. Let yourself relax completely now; let every muscle go loose and limp. Think of a very pleasant relaxing experience that you once had—maybe lying on the beach or crawling in between the sheets of your own bed when you were so tired and weary.

"You will notice a growing feeling of heaviness in your arm—perhaps a numbness. Your breathing is getting slower, deeper, and more regular. You are very much aware of what is going on around you, but you feel yourself going deeper and deeper relaxed with every breath you take. And if you really wish to go deeper, start counting backwards from one hundred to zero slowly. With every breath you take and every number you count backwards, you will go deeper, deeper, and still deeper relaxed.

"Let all your muscles relax still more completely. Begin with your feet . . . the right leg first. Let all the muscles relax—first those in your foot, then the ankle, the calf, and the upper leg. Now your left leg . . . from the toes to the hip. All right, now let your abdominal and stomach muscles relax, too. Let your chest and breathing muscles relax. Your shoulders, your arms, and your hands . . . relax all of them. Now your neck: let it relax. Do not mind if your head bows forward or to the side. It will be perfectly comfortable. Your facial muscles can relax, particularly the eyes and the lids. Relax completely . . . relax . . . every muscle in your body will relax.

"I am going to lift your hand now," the doctor will say; "let it rest lightly on my hand. Your arm and hand will soon lose the feeling of heaviness and will begin to grow lighter and lighter. In just a moment your hand will begin to lift up into the air without any voluntary effort on your part. Your arm, too, will get very light and start to lift, slowly but surely, up, up, upwards.

"It is so light now, without weight, as light as a feather. It seems as though it wants to move up, to lift upward, as though something is pulling it up. Now it is lifting up, away from my hand. That's right—up, up. Up higher—lifting higher and higher towards your face. Up . . . up. . . .

"As your arm lifts, you will go deeper and deeper relaxed. The higher your arms goes, the deeper relaxed you will go. And if you really wish to go deeper, your arm will rise higher. And if you wish to go still deeper, you will straighten your arm out, and the more rigid it gets, the deeper relaxed you will go. So just think and imagine, 'The stiffer my arm gets from my fingers to my shoulder, the deeper I'll go.'" (This is the catalepsy test that we mentioned earlier.)

At this point, you are in the cataleptic stage of hypnosis. You could keep your arm in this upraised position for an hour or more without feeling any discomfort—something you could not approach doing in a normal state of awareness. But your doctor is not interested in such theatrics, and he will relax you further as he directs you to lower your arm. "You will count backwards from ten to zero," he will say. "And, as you count, you will lower your arm with each number you count, and as your arm drops, you drop deeper relaxed—just as if you are on an escalator going down, down, and down. Ten . . . start lowering your arm and imagine that you are going deeper and deeper relaxed. Nine . . . each count takes you deeper. Eight . . . seven . . . six . . . still deeper. Five . . . four . . . three . . . you are now completely relaxed. Perhaps you might be willing to suggest to yourself that when your hands return to your lap, you will go deeper and deeper relaxed. Two . . . one . . . very deep now. And zero . . . you are very relaxed and perfectly comfortable. And as long as your arms remain comfortably relaxed in your lap—and with every breath you take—you'll go still deeper relaxed."

This is, in reality, "patient-oriented hypnosis".

CHAPTER V

•

Autohypnosis

"DAY BY DAY, in every way, I'm getting better and better."

Remember how you used to say this to yourself? Maybe you were trying to improve your mental health or physical skills, or to perfect a better memory, or just to develop a nicer personality. Repeating this simple sentence to yourself over and over again, particularly when you were younger, really did help most of the time. At least, you always felt better for trying it. This, indeed, is positive, constructive conditioning.

Well, while you are progressing with formal hypnotic training, your doctor will ask you to practice attaining deeper states of hypnosis at home by a method similar to the "day by day" system. We call this daily relaxation exercise "autohypnosis." With it, you will go through all the necessary steps to produce hypnosis just as you do when the doctor is inducing it. However, the only difference when you practice at home is that you will give these suggestions to yourself.

Aside from following your doctor's recommendations for physical care, practicing these relaxation exercises for inducing self-hypnosis is the most important thing you can do in the final weeks of your pregnancy to insure a pleasant, comfortable childbirth. For one thing, each time you hypnotize yourself, you will reduce the time required to reach deep hypnosis when either you or your doctor suggests it. You can see how valuable this training in autohypnosis will be if, for example, your physician is not immediately available when your labor begins. In fact, virtually all of our hypnotically-oriented patients arrive at the hospital for delivery in some stage of self-induced relaxation. Furthermore, even while you are developing a proficiency in relaxing yourself, you can utilize autohypnosis to eliminate some of the discomforts of pregnancy and to make "waiting" so much more pleasant. Far from being a chore, hypnotizing yourself will be something delightfully constructive to do with your time, and the actual effort will absorb no more than a few minutes in the morning and early evening each day.

The principles of autohypnosis are as old as hypnosis itself. Indeed, there is very little difference between the two because, as we have seen, even when the suggestions come from a hypnotist, in the end it is the subject who hypnotizes himself. This particular facet of hypnosis was especially fascinating to Emile Coué, a late-nineteenth-century French pharmacist and student of the power of suggestion. Coué reasoned that if subjects could be taught how to make constructive suggestions to themselves, they could realize all the benefits of hypnosis without going through the formalities of being hypnotized. In other words, heterohypnosis (involving two people—subject and operator) would be unnecessary.

Around the turn of the century, Coué established a school in his native country and taught his method of self-improvement—based upon the repetition of the "Day by day . . ." phrase—to literally thousands of pilgrims from Europe and the United States. At first, the results were astounding. The emotionally disturbed and even the physically ill who came back from France apparently cured by nothing more than suggestions that they gave themselves spread the pharmacist's fame far and wide. Children at school were taught the "Day by day . . ." pledge, and "Couéism" was proclaimed by many as a panacea for *all* of mankind's ills.

Unfortunately, Coué himself began to believe all of this

publicity. He undertook to cure ailments which only a trained physician could understand, and he began to work with less-imaginative patients, who found great difficulty in suggesting anything resembling a cure to themselves. News of the pharmacist's failures traveled as fast as had word of his earlier successes, and Couéism quickly slipped into the classification of a fad. Those vital ingredients for the induction of hypnosis—belief, faith, and *expectancy*— were missing.

Coué's techniques have long since lost their professional status. However, the dream of finding both an acceptable method of self-hypnosis and truly beneficial uses for the procedure continues to occupy other serious physicians, theologians, and writers. Mid-twentieth-century literature is full of books on "how you can help yourself to a better way of life." All over the world such new terms as autogenic training (in Germany), autoconditioning and progressive relaxation (in America), natural childbirth (in England), and conditioned reflexology and psychoprophylactic relaxation (in Russia and France) have been invented to describe some of the ancient Buddhist and Yoga teachings and the more contemporary dogmas of Christian Science and of "Divine healing," "the laying on of hands," and the "Royal Touch" of some evangelists and faith healers.

Autohypnosis has much in common with the state of prayer of many religions. All of the systems serve best the subject who is willing to devote a certain amount of time to daily practice in meditation, contemplation, introspection, and self-absorption—all of which are characterized by a concentration of awareness and, above all, by belief, confidence, and faith in the procedures. They all require a quiet, sedate atmosphere that is both free of distractions and conducive to a relaxed mind and body.

But autohypnosis is not a religion. Although its powers may seem truly amazing to those of us who have been operating on only a portion of our true capabilities, auto- hypnosis is not omnipotent. It cannot make you more bril- liant than the capacity of your brain will allow, or give you more physical strength than your muscular development permits, or enable you to bear pain above a very specific threshold or level. As a form of positive, constructive, health- ful conditioning, however, autohypnosis does enable you to go beyond your everyday abilities by almost anywhere from twenty to twenty-five per cent. What actually happens is that you tap your "forgotten assets," which you did not realize existed.

Very likely you have been doing this, under certain cir- cumstances, all your life. For instance, you could hang much longer from a tenth-floor window ledge if your life was at stake than you could from a gymnasium trapeze bar. Have you not been giving yourself autosuggestions all of your life without realizing it? Were you convinced that the first forkful of spinach you ever tasted would taste like sand? If so, it probably did. When you go to sleep at night, do you give yourself the suggestion that you will arise at a specific time in the morning? If you do, you may have wondered about the ability of your mind to keep time even while you are asleep. There are many other examples that we could cite of autosuggestions that, when repeated often enough and strongly enough, lead to autohypnosis. One of the more dramatic examples in everyday use con- cerns an old wives' tale, popular with some women a gener- ation or two ago, that the onset of menstruation could be delayed merely by twisting a thin red thread around the little finger of the left hand. Naturally, there was no scien- tific basis for this theory, but many women who *believed* that it would work were able to postpone the period for any time up to three days.

The big question, then, is not, "Will autohypnosis work?" Instead, the problem is *how* the subject can harness this innate ability or power that she has over herself. Can she turn it on and off, as she could water from a faucet, so that it will be there when she needs it—to control pain, for example? The answer is yes, if she will only follow a few simple rules and practice some techniques.

Your physician may suggest any one of many different methods for practicing autohypnosis. One technique, which was pioneered by a German psychiatrist, Dr. J. H. Schultz, and which is currently popular with many European physicians, is known as "autogenics." With this procedure, the subject begins to train herself by taking a comfortable seat in a quiet room at home. She lets her hands rest naturally in her lap, closes her eyes, and repeats to herself: "I am completely relaxed. . . . I am completely relaxed." She formulates this suggestion slowly and deliberately, pausing after each word.

The autogenic practice sessions should last only about a minute three times a day. At the conclusion of each period, the subject "alerts" herself by taking a deep breath and opening her eyes. That is all there is to it. After some weeks, Dr. Schultz claims, the subject should be able to relax herself at the very first suggestion. Then she can go on to give herself other beneficial suggestions.

She can, for instance, achieve a numbness (insensibility to pain) in any part of her body by doing little more than telling herself that numbness exists. After relaxing herself, the subject might merely repeat: "My left hand is getting numb. . . . My left hand is getting numb." After several weeks of practice, this effect, too, can be produced at the very first couple of suggestions, and the numbness can be transferred to any part of the body just by touching the numbed hand to that part. To remove all traces of numbness, the subject flexes the muscles of her hand and "alerts" herself as before.

Autogenics as a form of autohypnosis does work, if the subject wishes it to do so. The technique is useful in preparing the particularly resistant patient to accept hypnosis, in training her to break a bad habit, or in just teaching her how to relax. However, the weeks that a patient must spend in conditioning herself to accept suggestions with this method make it rather impractical for use in most obstetric cases.

Presently we shall discuss a more efficient procedure that you can use during your pregnancy. For the moment, the vital fact is that autohypnosis involves no more effort than that which we have just mentioned. Are you wondering, therefore, why, if autohypnosis is so simple, everyone does not use it to improve his golf game, to be more efficient at business, or to insure never—ever—suffering any pain? The answer is that practically all of these things and more are possible, but that, aside from overcoming an almost universal reluctance to practice, mankind must also rid itself of an exaggerated fear of the unknown. We think that, just because something cannot be fully explained at the moment, it must be forbidding. Did we not—not too long ago—believe that tomatoes were poisonous and that liver was inedible? Similarly, until now, because of their fears, men and women have been more the slaves than the masters of suggestion. A wise man once stated, "It is much easier to ignore the obvious than to renounce the traditional." This truism is valid today.

An interesting side light to this problem can be observed

in the rituals of some of the primitive tribes that still inhabit certain portions of the Old and New Worlds. In the Federation of Nigeria in Africa, for example, the inhabitants practice a form of autohypnosis that brings them very close, but not close enough, to the real advantages of suggestion. The natives hold endurance tests—called "sharos" —for young men, one of whom is flogged with an inch-thick stick by another. The object of the test is for the beaten one to prove his manliness by enduring the pain of the flogging without a trace of discomfort.

To accomplish this, the youth will hold a thorn in his mouth to prick his lips, dramatically demonstrating that the mind can "feel" but one pain at a time. He will also stare into a mirror or concentrate his attention elsewhere than on the pain of his wounds, so that even though the flogging raises angry welts, he will not cry out. Anthropologists have described couvade, in which the male goes through all the tortures of labor while his mate is having the baby free from all discomfort. Although we may question the reasons for these strange ceremonies, which have been going on for hundreds of years or more, we cannot deny that they, too, illustrate autosuggestion.

But we are not African bushmen; nor do most of us inflict physical pain upon ourselves needlessly. The "sharo" described above is important to us only because it dramatically demonstrates how far the body's endurance can be stretched with autohypnosis and how basically simple the procedure of giving oneself suggestions can be.

In our modern medical offices, you are not asked to perform any such senseless feats. Furthermore, you can practice your autohypnosis in the safe surroundings of your own home by giving yourself suggestions that you really wish to follow. The technique which your physician advises is both direct and easy to learn.

You begin by selecting a quiet room in the house and arranging to spend an uninterrupted half hour a day practicing there. Seated in a comfortable chair with your hands resting naturally in your lap and your feet squarely on the floor, you fix your eyes on a spot either on the ceiling overhead or on a point on the wall above the level of your eyes.

Then you commence counting to yourself slowly from one to ten. You direct your attention to your eyelids and, between numbers, tell yourself repeatedly that your eyelids are getting very, very heavy and that your eyes are getting very, very tired. Over and over again you say: "My lids are getting so heavy. I will feel as if I want to close my eyes at the count of three. My lids are getting heavier and heavier. I can just feel my lids getting so heavy, and the heavier they get, the deeper relaxed I will become and the better able I will be to follow all suggestions I give myself. Now my lids are getting very heavy. It's going to feel so good to close my eyes."

Do not be afraid to talk to yourself—and, above all, do not be afraid to listen. Some patients find it more efficient to say the words out loud; others prefer to "think" the words. In any case, you will find it a rewarding experience to "mind yourself" for a change, especially when you discover that what you are saying makes sense.

By the time you count to two, give yourself enough suggestions like the ones just mentioned so that you actually "feel" the heaviness of your eyelids. When you are sure that your lids are indeed heavy, count to three and let your eyes roll up into the back of your head for a few seconds. Then say to yourself: "My lids are now locked so tight that I doubt very much that I can open them. My lids shut tighter and tighter, and as my lids lock tight, I begin to feel a nice, calm, soothing, relaxed feeling beginning in my toes, moving into my legs and into my thighs—as I keep counting. It's the same feeling that I have in my jaws when my dentist injects novocain into them—the same feeling that I have when I fall asleep on my arm—the same feeling that I have when I sit too long in one position—the identical feeling that I would have in my legs if I sat cross-legged on them. A numb, woodenlike feeling starting in my toes is beginning to move up, up, up from my toes into my legs."

Next, count to four and say to yourself: "By the time I have counted to five, my legs from my toes to my thighs will be just as heavy as lead. I can feel my legs relaxing from my toes to my thighs. I can feel them getting heavier and heavier and heavier. Five: they are so heavy now that I don't think I can move them." Then double back for purposeful repetition. "My eyelids are locked tight, so tight that I don't believe I can open them. My legs from my toes to my thighs are completely relaxed." Each time you re-trace these autosuggestions, you stamp in the learned response pattern.

You continue in this way: "By the time I have counted to six and seven, my fingers, hands, and arms will be very, very heavy. I am beginning to feel that same numbness moving up from my fingers to my shoulders. A heavy, detached feeling is moving up from my fingers to my hand, to my wrist, past my elbows, up to my arm, to my shoulder. Both my arms, from my hands to my shoulders, are getting very numb—a heavy, woodenlike numbness. When I have counted to seven, my arms will be just as heavy and relaxed as my eyelids, and as numb as my legs, are now."

Do not worry if you forget the exact words. They are

far less important than the effect that you are trying to achieve—a feeling of numbness all the way from the finger tips to the wrist, to the elbow, to the shoulder, to the neck. In practice, this may be a bit more difficult to accomplish in the first few sessions at home, but the feeling will come faster in subsequent attempts. It is most important that you never become discouraged and that you not tire yourself by spending more than the half hour a day in practice.

When you finally reach the point where, by the count of seven, your limbs are sufficiently relaxed, you repeat again all the suggestions you have given yourself, adding: "My legs are so heavy that I don't believe I can move them. My eyes are locked so tight that I doubt that I can open them. My arms are so heavy that I cannot lift them, and by the time I have counted from seven to eight, my trunk will be relaxed."

Now go back to the lids, legs, and arms. Then say: "By the time I count from eight to nine, my chest will have relaxed, too. With every breath I take, I can just feel myself going deeper and deeper into a relaxed state. My back and abdomen are getting very, very numb. I can feel the muscles in my chest relaxing. Eight: my entire body, from my neck down, is relaxed. Nine: I am completely relaxed. . . . I can't open my eyes. . . . I can't move my legs. . . . I can't move my arms. I feel my whole body relaxed, thoroughly and deeply. It is so refreshing to remain in this deep, quiet state.

"I will now relax my neck and head, so that, at the count of ten, I will be completely relaxed from my head to my toes. I can feel that with every breath I take I am becoming calmer and deeper relaxed . . . deeper and deeper relaxed . . . into a calm, soothing, refreshing state. Everything is just getting more and more relaxed. I feel as if I am floating away . . . falling deeper and deeper . . . not asleep, but just thoroughly relaxed. Ten: I am completely relaxed. My eyes and limbs are as heavy as lead. My entire body feels numb, heavy, woodenlike, as I go deeper and deeper."

Success! You have now hypnotized yourself by going from the smallest muscles of the body—the lids—to increasingly larger ones, such as toes, fingers, trunk, and chest. This is indeed "progressive relaxation." Now it is only logical that you should ask: "What can I do with this new ability I have just developed?" Well, for one thing, there is the rather obvious fact that you have achieved a point of outward calm and inner peace that you could not reach in a normal state of awareness with its thousand and one distractions. In addition, everything you will learn to do with hypnosis can be duplicated with autohypnosis. Of course, the specific effects that you will be able to reproduce will depend upon how deeply you hypnotize yourself. Your degree of susceptibility to suggestions that you may give yourself will increase as you go from the hypnoidal stages towards the somnambulistic stages, just as it does with hypnosis.

Among all the uses to which you will put autohypnosis, one of the most rewarding will be the posthypnotic suggestions that you implant in your mind. For instance, you can shorten the time for subsequent autohypnosis by the use of time distortion—telling yourself that twenty minutes will seem like one minute. Does this not happen when time passes rapidly, as during a good movie or lecture? Further relaxation can be obtained by giving yourself the suggestion that when you think of a color (soothing green, perhaps), you will instantly become relaxed. You may select any color or any other signal that comes to you naturally.

After you have taught yourself how to relax, you can practice the development of glove anesthesia and learn how to transfer that effect to your abdomen and other parts of your body. The only restrictions in utilizing autohypnosis are that you select a word or sign which is short and direct and that you employ it only in a safe and secure environment. When you do that, there is no more danger that you will accidentally hypnotize yourself than there is that you can be hypnotized against your will.

Much has been written about the proper form of posthypnotic suggestions that a subject can give to herself. Undoubtedly, your physician will want to make a few recommendations of his own. This is because the phrasing of the suggestions, for best results, will depend upon your own background, education, and anxieties. Remember, though, your autohypnosis will not depend upon any special schooling. No matter how you say things, as an obstetric patient all of your practice sessions—after you have been relaxed during the autohypnotic state—should include suggestions similar to the following:

"I will look forward to having my baby with a feeling of joy and happiness. I will not have the slightest dread or anticipation of unhappiness. I will be able to relax during the height of the uterine contractions. I will look forward, too, to being fully alert and completely aware or conscious when my baby is born. I'd love to hear the first cry of my baby, because I want to feel the continuity of the entire birth process. I do not want to have any disruption or gap occur."

In order to terminate the autohypnotic state instantaneously, all you have to do is to think to yourself, "One: I'll go deeper relaxed the next time I try this. Two: I'll follow all of the suggestions I have given to myself to the

best of my ability. Three: I'll open my eyes and feel fine—
wonderful."

This type of suggestion, if repeated often enough during
the prenatal period, will be valuable whether or not you
can achieve deep hypnosis during labor and delivery. After
all, there is no guarantee that because you are a particularly
good subject in the office, at group sessions, and at home,
you will also be completely comfortable in childbirth. But
there is no doubt that your discomfort will be greatly
diminished if you practice your autohypnosis lessons faithfully.

One of our patients, Mrs. B.C., a woman in her late
forties expecting her second child, was particularly resistant
to hypnosis, even during her prenatal training. Putting her
personal anxieties aside, she attended every group class
and did not become discouraged with her futile attempts
at autohypnosis. She practiced regularly and repeated her
suggestions to herself at each session. At childbirth she had
a relatively short and painless labor, and she felt no pain
whatsoever in delivering until the crowning of the head
occurred. No anesthesia was needed for the episiotomy,
delivery, and repair. No analgesia was used at any time
during the labor. This patient's composure—and the smooth
course of her labor—could be attributed only to the prenatal
conditioning in autohypnosis.

A younger patient, Mrs. Y.B., was most desirous of
experiencing "painless labor" with hypnosis, and she made
an excellent subject during her prenatal period. Yet, in
the delivery room, she resisted deep relaxation because
she wished to "see, hear, and feel everything" during this,
her first, delivery. Nevertheless, in spite of very hard contractions and a protracted labor of thirty-six hours, she reported "no pain," even when an extremely deep episiotomy

was performed. And during its repair she played with her newborn infant and felt nothing but a sense of happiness.

Such cases are examples of a phenomenon that is closely related to autohypnosis and is called "waking hypnosis." By this we mean the ability of a subject to respond to suggestions (even when she gives them herself) given while she is in a normal state of awareness. We have already observed simpler instances of this type of hypnosis—for example, the case of the wave of coughing that can be heard in any theater audience after just one person has cleared his throat. This, as you will remember from Chapter III, is called an "ideomotor" reaction.

Bear in mind that none of these individuals is consciously aware of following suggestions. Although we do not know exactly why the phenomenon of autohypnosis occurs, we recognize that whenever individuals think the same thoughts over and over again, they sort of "sales-talk" themselves into a fixed idea. And the critical attitudes are not mobilized as readily against an idea when the thoughts originate from the subject herself. This partly explains the power of all persons to accept some autosuggestions without going through formal hypnosis. When these suggestions affect our senses (alleviating pain, for example), they induce what are called "ideosensory" reactions; when they induce involuntary responses, such as the back-seat driver's "stepping on the brakes," they are called, as we have stated, "ideomotor" reactions.

Certainly the deeper the hypnosis, the better the results; but to a degree you will be able to stimulate ideosensory and ideomotor responses in yourself just by imagining certain suggestions over and over again. You can control some pain just as easily by imagining a pleasant experience as you can make your mouth "water" by thinking of a delicious meal. If you make the suggestion often enough, the response will be just as instantaneous as an involuntary cough. This is what we mean when we say that autohypnosis can be useful to the obstetric patient even if she never achieves deeper hypnosis.

The most important point to remember in autohypnosis, then, is to be consistent. It is also necessary to give yourself suggestions via the imagination rather than the will. Remember that "imagination power" is more potent than will power. For instance, you cannot *will* your mouth to water, but if you imagine a past pleasant mealtime experience, your mouth will drool readily. Finally, you should make it a habit to include two specific suggestions in each session. First, you should tell yourself exactly what procedure you will use to "alert" yourself. (More about this follows in just a moment.) Second, as has been mentioned, you should terminate each practice period with the autosuggestion that the next time autohypnosis is attempted the result will be swifter and deeper hypnosis.

We wish to emphasize that the procedure for dehypnotizing yourself is the simplest imaginable. At the risk of belaboring the point, we stress that you merely have to tell yourself that you will count from one through three and give yourself a few "alerting" suggestions along the way. At the count of one, you say that you feel wonderful—no headache, no numbness, just health and happiness—and that you will have no untoward effects from the experience. With two, you suggest that you will open your eyes promptly at the count of three. Then you say—and remember that this may be either silently or aloud—that you will go into a deeper and more profound state of relaxation the next time you hypnotize yourself: "I will continue to practice and, with each successive hypnotic induction, I will become deeper and deeper relaxed." Finally, you count to three, take a deep breath, exhale, and open your eyes. The autohypnotic state will have been terminated.

You can use this state for relieving fear, anxiety, or tension; for eliminating or reducing fatigue; for accelerating your ability to fall asleep; and for improving your memory and concentration.

We have never seen the slightest danger from the use of autohypnosis; and no one has ever failed to come out of it. Anyone who can induce it can also most certainly terminate it. There is, in reality, no fine line of separation between autosuggestion and autohypnosis—one merges into the other. And these states occur continually at nonhypnotic levels. We are all continually going in and out of reverie-like states, as in daydreaming, depersonalization, and the complete detachment that is characteristic of the preoccupation with other more urgent and pressing thoughts. The only theoretical danger lies in giving this ability to a person who already is detached or depersonalized. No physician would think of pushing an individual who is already "out of this world" into a state of autohypnosis. Nor would he allow an individual who spends a great deal of time in autistic thinking or introspection to learn all about autohypnosis.

We wish to point out, therefore, that the above suggestions for autohypnotic development *can and should be taught only* by your physician. They are achieved only after heterohypnosis has been induced—and that should be induced by a doctor, not by you or a layman.

Autohypnosis should have a salutary effect, and it should make childbirth a more satisfying procedure that can and will fulfill deep, but often unrecognized and unformulated, needs in the mother. Given wisely and judiciously by a qualified physician, training in autohypnosis can be a boon to all mothers-to-be.

CHAPTER VI

·

Hypnosis and Pain

HONESTY OF PURPOSE is essential to successful hypnosis. The faddist, who, as we have said, is tempted to try hypnosis because she will be the first in her crowd to do so, quickly loses both her interest and her ability to concentrate. No doctor on earth can do much with such an individual. Her inability to direct her attention fully to the task at hand makes her highly resistant to hypnosis, and that, in turn, causes her attention span to be decreased. It is a vicious cycle that can be broken only by the subject's reapplying herself to following suggestions.

On the other hand, the person who is truthful with herself and who approaches motherhood highly motivated to have a baby has very little difficulty in maintaining her practice sessions. It may be argued that this purposeful fixation for hypnosis is, in itself, a form of hypnosis. That may be so, but the more important point to remember is that such goal-directed thoughts are to be found only in the best and happiest subjects.

If you are like the vast majority of patients, you have sought out hypnosis because you are afraid of the pains that you associate with childbirth. This is even more likely if you are pregnant with your first child or if you are experienced in the role of becoming a mother but your earlier deliveries were complicated and painful.

There is certainly nothing abnormal about such fears; nor is it our intention to dismiss these fears lightly with the statement that the pains commonly associated with childbirth are "all in your mind." For, as we shall presently discover, these pains are very real indeed. In fact, the entire subject of pain is so complex and pertinent to our discussion that we have divided it into two parts. The first, covered by this chapter, will deal with the true origin of most pain.

The second, reserved for Chapter VII, concerns the role that hypnosis plays in alleviating pain.

Pain is necessary for protective purposes. It is often a signal of danger. Therefore, some pain is inescapable. And truly, we would not want it any other way. Imagine a life free of all pain! It would certainly be pleasant enough, but we would have no warning of organic disorders, and physical disaster would overtake us before we were even aware that anything was wrong. For example, persistent headaches during pregnancy may indicate a toxic condition with a rising blood pressure and should be called to the attention of your obstetrician as soon as possible. You should also call your doctor about chills accompanied by a rise in temperature, persistent dizziness, or any other disturbing symptom, particularly during pregnancy.

Such distresses *could* be due to some part of your body's going awry. They are the sorts of things which result from either an inadequate diet or a definite physical lack. When such a deficiency makes a patient ill, we refer to her complaint as an organic or "structural" one, and we proceed to strengthen her body with modern drugs and medicines.

However, twentieth-century medicine accepts the fact that sometimes there is no physical reason for the failure of a body to function properly. As a case in point, bladder trouble is not necessarily an indication of a diseased kidney. We are also unable to detect any physical breakdown in the hay fever sufferer. Still, there is a malfunctioning of some segment of the patient in each of these instances.

The study of why structurally healthy organs produce genuine symptoms of disease and also cause pain is known as "psychosomatics." Broadly speaking, this word, derived from the Greek "psyche," which once meant breath, refers to *the interaction of our emotions and other mental proc-*

esses with physical factors to influence our body's performance. In other words, although we may be really sick and have actual pains and aches, the root of our difficulties is more mental than physical. The list of psychosomatic illnesses is already quite large and is growing with each passing day of research. It already includes colitis, migraine headaches, peptic ulcers, obesity, asthma, allergies, menstrual disturbances, and other female disorders. We should especially note that many discomforts of pregnancy, such as nausea and vomiting, and of difficulty in labor and delivery in normally healthy women are also known to be psychosomatic in origin.

You are probably wondering, "Can our thoughts really make us ill and cause us to suffer pain even against our will?" This question has occupied many of the finest medical minds in the world, and their conclusion is that we are actually no healthier or free from discomfort than we think we are.

During World War II, Dr. Henry K. Beecher of Harvard University compared the reactions to pain of one hundred fifty wounded soldiers on the Anzio beachhead battleground in Italy with those of a like number of male civilian surgical patients in the United States. "The striking thing about the war wounds, and the men involved," Dr. Beecher stated, "was their comparative freedom from pain." Only one quarter of the entire group of badly-wounded servicemen, when questioned seven to twelve hours after being wounded, had enough pain to want anything done about it. On the other hand, more than eighty per cent of the civilian patients, when interviewed an average of less than four hours after surgery, had pain severe enough to request a narcotic.

Dr. Beecher concluded: "In a situation in which a wound

has great advantage, and means escape from overpowering anxiety and fear of death on the battlefield (as in the case of war wounds terminating military service), extensive wounds are associated with comparatively little pain. In a situation in which the wound connotes disaster (for example, major surgery in civil life), lesser wounds are associated with far more pain than in the former situation. *The essential difference appears to be in the difference in anxiety level in the two cases, in the attitude of the patient, and in his reaction to his wound."*

From such research as Dr. Beecher's, we have learned a great deal about why no two patients perceive pain in exactly the same manner—even on such a common meeting ground as the hospital delivery room. Physicians, who long ago observed that some women experience more pain in labor than others, now recognize that sudden and violent emotions of the mind have a powerful influence on the contractions of the uterus. Indeed, with no other apparent cause, the contractions of the patient may be completely suspended, or their energy may be greaty impaired—and in either case the result is discomfort and pain.

Before plunging headlong into the subjects of where these emotions come from and what we can do about controlling them, let us consider how we feel pain. It will help if you keep the classic image of the brain as a switchboard in front of you. It is a fact that a network of nerves, far more complicated than any communications system devised by man, conducts impulses in and out of this "switchboard."

Let us assume that you have just struck your finger with a hammer. At the risk of oversimplification, we can say that the free nerve endings just below the surface of your skin will pick up this physical stimulus and transmit it, via the "somatic" nerve network and the spinal cord, to the pain reception centers of your brain. There, a second signal, which we call a "motor response," will be transmitted back to the muscles of your hand so that you will almost instantly pull back from the source of danger and pain. So efficient is this built-in communications network of yours that the time lapse between stimulus and response will probably be no more than 1/1000th of a second.

If we consider next a simple but frightening emotional stimulus, such as the sight of a speeding automobile bearing down upon us, we will realize that our "switchboard" can be alerted just as effectively by a thought. Naturally, we are afraid that the auto will hit us, and so we seem to leap spontaneously from its path. But in that fraction of a second between the time we first sense the danger and the time we respond to it, the trunk lines of our network are busy transmitting messages back and forth over sympathetic pathways of the nervous system. The result is a marshaling of all of nature's forces to meet the danger.

Take, for example, the individual who "runs for his life": he runs faster than even he ever thought possible. The source for this extra ounce of energy, triggered by an emotional impulse in the brain, is the endocrine system of glands in the body. You are probably already familiar with the names of a few of these glands, such as the thyroid, adrenal, and pancreas. All of them manufacture chemical substances known as hormones which, when ejected into the blood stream, individually alter the sugar content or temperature of the body so that we are physically capable of responding to certain stimuli. In the case of the oncoming auto, these chemicals enable our legs to carry us to safety speedily.

The benefits of being able to "run" from some distressing situations are obvious. We all encounter such stimuli every day of our lives. However, there are times when we either cannot or do not want to run, and it is these moments which are filled with pain-provoking possibilities. The woman who approaches childbirth with fear of pain, for example, may subconsciously or even consciously wish to run from the situation. But her uterus cannot fly from its own activities: it can only respond with resistance to the nerve impulses stimulated by that fear. It does this by contracting, or tightening, certain muscles at its "neck" and around its lower segments. As the fear is intensified, the motor responses of the woman are magnified and the resistance is increased. Naturally, the greater the muscular contraction, the greater the force required for dilation, and the greater the stimulus to the pain receptors in the uterus itself. The patient, sensing this pain, can then think only that her original fears were justified. Thus, we have an unfortunate cycle of fear, tension, and pain that can cause extreme discomfort and difficulty in an otherwise uncomplicated labor.

Of course, it is theoretically possible to break this vicious cycle at either the fear, tension, or pain level. Chemical anesthesia is most effective in removing physical pain from childbirth. However, the mental route for transmission of pain is still open. But hypnosis can effectively block the mental perception of pain, and it is here that the technique has its greatest usefulness. In the following chapter, we shall discover how simply hypnosis can alleviate our fears and tensions. But hypnosis works best when the subject is fully aware of what the doctor is trying to accomplish. Therefore, if you can understand where your emotions originate, your hypnosis will be even more successful.

First of all, we should explain that although we have been discussing only the emotion of fear, there are many other mental states which can influence the way you "feel" at the moment. Love, hatred, disgust, pride, anger, and sadness are just a few of the numerous emotions to which the mind is heir. All of them will play some role in your reaction to the birth process. Still, that reaction will never be exactly the same for you as it is for any other woman, because your responses will vary according to your background and upbringing.

Freud tells us that a person's personality pattern, or the sum of her reactions to her past experiences, is developed in several early stages occurring from birth to five or six years of age. In the first, or "oral," stage he includes all forms of sensual gratification, such as nursing and thumb-sucking. This stage, Freud says, is characterized chiefly by desires which make the mouth the most excitable zone and which satisfy the infant's emotional and physical needs. Repeated frustration of these oral demands, as in the case of too long a wait between feedings, results in anxiety and tension. The baby reacts to these with rage, typified at first by crying and later by biting. Even though the parents eventually "get the message" and satisfy the child's physical demands, psychiatrists maintain, the imprint on the personality has been made, and it may later return in the form of certain adult character traits, such as greediness and disgust.

The second, or "anal," period of the infant, according to Freud, is noticeable by the pleasurable excitation of the anal zone resulting from either the passage or the withholding of the feces. Cruel, sadistic, or miserly tendencies can arise in later life, we are told, if this stage of development is mishandled: for example, too early or too rigid toilet training can result in withholding tendencies.

It is fairly common for this personality trait of the infant to make itself known in the delivery room. We observe it frequently in the case of a woman whose uterine contractions are inhibited by an emotional voyage back to her own infancy: the patient's pelvic muscles are unable to contract because of her lifelong unwillingness to give up products emanating from her own body. Such women cannot even secrete milk from their breasts even though they are milk-laden.

Although authorities differ as to when we first learn to respond emotionally, there is no doubt that our lessons begin before we reach the peak of our physical development. For this reason, you will find physicians attaching great importance to knowing not only how the patient passed through the Freudian stages of infantile sexuality but also how she approached the climactic changes of puberty, adolescence, marriage, and motherhood. In some women the effects of emotions on their reproductive functions are expressed as menstrual disorders, frigidity, and infertility long before they ever become pregnant.

Sometimes our search to isolate the emotion which is inhibiting labor and delivery takes us into strange corners of the mind. For one thing, there is an undeniable although unconscious pleasure that many women find in pain. As a matter of fact, quite a few candidates for motherhood feel duty-bound to endure "labor pains" stoically. This "pleasure in displeasure" is known as self-suffering or masochism; more often than not, however, it is simply the result of a misunderstanding of what is expected of the woman in labor. There is, too, the feeling of self-love, very apparent in many patients, which rebels against anything that threatens the person's physical or mental comfort. The psychologist's word for this emotion, in the extreme, is "narcissism", but it is obvious that all individuals harbor narcissistic tendencies to a degree. In fact, the very essence of womanhood is a blending of these qualities.

Very likely, the root for this sensation in a woman can be found in the adolescent years. At that time, the young female abandons most of her childlike attempts to gain parental approval and strikes out for greener pastures. She begins to sense newly-developed sexual drives and wishes to be "loved." Society, however, frowns upon "boy-chasing" —the logical outlet for her drives, which no longer find satisfaction in parental love. Therefore, in her search for a socially acceptable outlet, the adolescent turns to self-love. Thus, she preserves both her self-confidence and her self-respect.

We could go on to explore all the other emotions which can influence a woman's behavior and sensations in childbirth, but we would find none so universal as fear. Therefore, let us dwell for a while upon the origins of fears and upon the odd forms that they assume even in this enlightened civilization of ours.

We can recall a well-meaning nurses' aide who, while she took patients up to the delivery floor, would remark: "You poor darling, I feel so sorry for you. I suffered so much when I had my baby." The damage created was so obvious that the woman was soon transferred to another station. Unfortunately, we cannot remove all causes of fear so easily.

We can safely assume that the fears of the average woman in the delivery room are much deeper than just the fear of chemical anesthesia. For instance, sometimes a woman develops an identification with the fetus during pregnancy. As a result, she is reluctant to give up this strong emotional attachment to the fetus, which she fancies as an inseparable part of her body. As separation becomes imminent, the patient may develop profound anxiety and fear over the impending loss of a "part of myself." Sometimes this is expressed as: "I felt much better when I was carrying the child than I do now that he is born." Of course, this reasoning takes place in the subconscious area, where it cannot be attacked by the logic of the attending physician; but the fear it generates is none the less real.

In quite a few cases, the fear of the patient is less for herself and more for her husband or child. A typical example of how this type of fear can interfere with the birth process very early in pregnancy may be seen in the following brief history of one of our patients.

Mrs. V.W., aged twenty-nine years, was admitted to the hospital in her third month of pregnancy with a history of severe nausea and vomiting accompanied by abdominal pain. This obviously ill woman was extremely nervous and weak and complained of headaches. In spite of all the usual therapy—consisting of dietary restrictions, sedation, etc.—the vomiting persisted until, one day, deep hypnosis was induced.

Posthypnotic suggestions that she would have no more nausea and vomiting and that she would look forward to having her baby with a feeling of joy and happiness were given to the patient while she was in the hypnotic state. The result was a complete and dramatic cessation of the symptoms. This woman was able to eat her regular diet from that day on, and she left the hospital in excellent physical condition. She later revealed that she had not desired the pregnancy because of her poor financial condition and the possibility that she might separate from her husband.

From the standpoint of both the doctor and the expectant mother, the worst part about such fears is that although they are present in almost every maternity case, they defy analysis and treatment by remaining below the surface of conscious awareness. Every emotionally healthy woman will tell you that she truly *wants* a child for any one of a number of apparently good reasons—a desire to make a happy home, a method of gratifying her mate, the production of an object for the investment of her own love and interest, an heir to the family name, or the grateful fulfillment of her obligation to society.

Yet obstetricians know that behind each of these admirable reasons for wanting a child are many fears that stifle the natural chain of events culminating in childbirth. Depending upon the emotional maturity of the woman, these could be fear of the child's being born deformed, mentally or physically; fear of death to the child; fear of the pains of childbirth; fear of "getting out of shape"; and fear of the responsibility of bringing up a child.

But we have still not mentioned the biggest fear of all. This, the psychologists say, is the most common of all the emotions. "In all women," they tell us, "the happy and the disappointed, the strong and the weak, the loving and the hating—the doubts, restlessness, impatience and joyful expectation, all conceal the fear of delivery. And all these fears are only provocations, or intensifications of a deep hereditary fear of death."

Naturally, in these days when giving birth to a child is no more dangerous for the mother than the most minor surgery, such fears are absolutely groundless. Still, they persist in a majority, if not in all, of the women we meet. We might also add that this overconcern with death is hardly confined to the female of the species. Men and women, young and old, rich and poor—all of mankind is so obsessed with thoughts of death that the anxiety spills over into such everyday phrases as "cut him *dead*" or "stop him *dead* in his tracks" without the speaker's quite realizing what he is saying.

We also seldom realize the price we pay in discomfort for these subconscious thoughts. The idea of death, for even the most courageous of us, is always accompanied by anxiety. Reconsider, for a moment, the example mentioned earlier of an automobile hurtling down the road towards you. Surely you may be expected to respond with fear in this situation. But this fear, we discovered, is good, because it stimulates your glands into supplying you with the blood chemicals you need to leap out of harm's way swiftly.

But suppose that instead of just one car, there were two—approaching in opposite directions. You would not know which way to jump, would you? Chances are that you would start to perspire. The muscles around the pit of your stomach would become tense, and perhaps you would even feel faint. In short, you would be displaying all of the classic symptoms of anxiety—and with good reason, you would be sure, because your life was being threatened. But the valuable lesson here is that none of these responses to danger could possibly save you. Rather, they would probably make you "sick" even after the threat had passed.

There is nothing to be gained from anxiety—except, perhaps, ulcers in the case of the insecure executive who feels that his business "existence" is threatened or migraine headaches in the case of the envious mother who believes that her family wishes her "out of the way." These expressions, of course, are due to guilty fears over their hostile and aggressive impulses. In cases of childbirth, women often reveal this same concern by expressing the fear that the baby might "kill" the beautiful relationship between themselves and their husbands. The subterfuges of their true emotions are many, but the results are always more difficulties in labor than are necessary.

It is difficult to say exactly when death first becomes associated with childbirth in a woman's mind. Obviously, the harrowing tales of difficult deliveries related by well-meaning friends and relatives play some part in formulating such thoughts. But nothing that she can hear in adult life can impress a woman more than what she hears in her own mother-daughter relationship.

When the mother attempts to win respect from her child by relating how much she "suffered" to bring her into the world, she is laying the groundwork for painful emotions and unpleasant sensations in her daughter's labors. Considering the tales that some women tell their children to gain respect and admiration, it is no wonder that these youngsters in later years are "scared to death" of childbirth.

CHAPTER VII

•

Alleviating Pain with Hypnosis

WITH HYPNOSIS YOU may control pain in any one of a number of ways. If you know, for example, that you are about to enter a painful situation, you may relax yourself beforehand and give yourself the suggestion that you will feel no pain in that situation. The effectiveness of this posthypnotic suggestion, whether it is initiated by you or your physician, depends upon the depth of hypnosis achieved and upon the severity of the pain. If you practice long and hard enough, you may eventually be able to duplicate the feats of the Indian fakirs who can sit upon beds of nails or walk across glowing coals with no apparent discomfort. Interesting as it may be to think about these extreme examples of the power of suggestion, the modern American housewife has little need for such talents. Besides conditioning himself to accept such suggestions, the fakir must spend so much time in practice that he takes a vow of poverty to rid himself of such petty considerations as earning a living. This vow is obviously no concern of a woman who is interested primarily in comfortable childbirth.

We have already touched upon another method by which you may, if you are a good subject, alleviate pain with hypnosis. That is the use of hypnotic amnesia. If you really wish to do so, you can forget everything that happened to you, everything you heard, and every sensation you experienced while you were hypnotized. Therefore, while you may be uncomfortable in a painful situation, if you enter it in a deeply relaxed frame of mind, when it is all over you do not have to remember how you felt. The mere suggestion that you will forget will be sufficient to erase the experience from your memory. You can also be taught how to use another phenomenon of hypnosis—time distortion. By such measures, you will have no concept of the passage of time. Hours of labor, for instance, will seem to be no more than a minute.

Undoubtedly, you had many similar experiences long before you became pregnant or ever heard of hypnosis. Perhaps you can recall standing on a street corner and waiting for a bus while chatting pleasantly with a friend. Remember how swiftly the time seemed to pass? Conversely, the minutes seemingly stretched into hours when you waited alone on the corner in foul weather.

Hypnotic amnesia and time distortion, which are merely the formalization of everyday experiences, have a very real role to play in medicine. Their use in hypnotherapy involving the treatment of certain psychosomatic disorders cannot be disputed. But the most cherished moment in the lives of many women is the memory of childbirth. Hypnosis need not blot out the details of that experience. Indeed, one of the very real benefits of the procedure is that it brings childbirth into sharper focus so that the mother is always fully aware of the contribution she has made.

For all of these reasons, we prefer to alleviate the pain of our patients/subjects not by striking it from their memories but by altering their emotional reactions to it. Surely, even in a deep somnambulistic state, a woman may know that she is experiencing pain in her abdomen and pelvic region if there is some physical basis for the fact. But the pain is not perceived as pain (in the commonly accepted sense of that word) by the portion of the brain which interprets these signals. That is to say, the patient is aware of the pain and will remember it; however, instead of being annoying or downright uncomfortable, the pain will be just another indicator of the immensely satisfying childbirth experience. This is what we mean when we say that with hypnosis we may change the patient's perception of pain.

To see how this works practically, let us consider again the report of Dr. Beecher, whose research on the reactions of individuals to pain was mentioned in the preceding chapter. The doctor noted that the mere suggestion of relief was sufficient to inhibit the spread of painful impulses in many of his patients. Over twenty per cent of these persons reported "considerable" relief after receiving placebos, or inert chemicals which could not possibly have had any alleviating effect—unless the patient wished it. His subjects, Dr. Beecher stated, did not claim that pain was absent. Rather, they appeared to be mentally divorced from painful experience. In other words, the pain was there, but it no longer bothered them.

You may attain this same satisfying state with hypnosis. Your physician will, no doubt, instruct you how to do this with a widely-used phenomenon of hypnosis known as "glove anesthesia," which we mentioned earlier. After you have reached one of the deeper stages of hypnosis and are resting comfortably with your hands once more naturally in your lap, he will suggest that you again think of one hand.

"Concentrate on that hand," he will say. "As you think about it, very hard, you will notice a tingling sensation in your finger tips. First, it will be the tip of just one finger—a heavy, insensitive spot, small at first, but gradually spreading into a larger numb area. Notice that numblike feeling moving slowly, but steadily, up the finger and into the hand.

"Now you are feeling the same thing in other fingers of that hand—a very heavy sensation . . . something like the last time your hand fell asleep. Remember how that felt.

. . . Your entire hand is now numb, very numb. You can feel the heaviness moving up the fingers, up the palm, and up to your wrist. Imagine, if you will, that you have put on a glove and that underneath that glove the entire hand is getting more and more numb, heavy, and woodenlike.

"All right now, if you really wish to transfer that same numb feeling and insensibility to any part of your body, you may do so easily. All you have to do is touch your hand to that part and leave it there until the heavy feeling flows from your hand into that part of you which you want to make numb. It is so easy to do. . . . You can make any segment of your body heavy and completely deadened to pain. After you are certain that all the numbness has flowed from your hand into this area, you will remove your hand, which will feel quite normal; but the part that you touched will be so numb that you will feel no pain."

In less time than it took for you to read the last couple of paragraphs, you can "anesthetize" any part of your body just by following such suggestions. Of course, you will have to reach the cataleptic stage of hypnosis, at least, before you can induce this hypnoanesthesia. Also, very probably it will not be possible for you to do much more than make your finger tips numb in the first couple of attempts. But each time you induce anesthesia, it will cover a larger area until, eventually, the entire imaginary "glove" will be numb and you will be able to transfer this numbness to other parts of your body. To speed up the process, your physician will ask you to practice inducing this anesthesia in your daily sessions with autohypnosis at home.

Hypnosis as an adjunct to reduce the amount of anesthesia is here! It has reduced the need for drugs and anesthesia in thousands of deliveries, and all sorts of major surgery have been performed with its aid in many reputable hospitals across the land. Therefore, for the physician trained in this technique, the average delivery with hypnosis is a comparatively simple affair. In 1956 the author participated with Dr. Sol T. DeLee in a Caesarean section delivery and hysterectomy at the Chicago Lying-in Hospital that illustrates how effective hypnosis can be even in cases of unusual delivery.

Our patient was a married woman, twenty-seven years of age, who had twice before given birth via Caesarean section. In each of those instances, chemicals and drugs were used to induce anesthesia. This time, however, she expressed a strong wish to participate fully in the entire experience. For this reason—and because of her extreme apprehension concerning the use of chemoanesthesia (inhalation, spinal, or "local")—it was decided to perform the entire operation using pure hypnosis, if possible. As near as we can determine, this was the first operation of its kind ever performed with hypnosis.

Around the beginning of the seventh month of her pregnancy, this patient was hypnotized for the first time. A few weeks earlier, susceptibility tests had indicated that she would, indeed, make an excellent subject. As a matter of fact, it was only necessary to hypnotize her a total of six times before she was able to exhibit most of the phenomena of deep hypnosis—particularly anesthesia and the abilities to follow posthypnotic suggestions and to enter into complete rapport with the operator. Because of this, she quickly learned the techniques of autohypnosis and could develop hypnoanesthesia by following suggestions for pain relief that she either gave herself or was given by the hypnotist.

During one of these sessions prior to the operation, all of the details of the operation itself were described to the patient while she was in a deep hypnotic state. This dress rehearsal of each step in surgery, including everything except the actual incision, is a common technique with hypnoanesthesia. Furthermore, most physicians will attempt to make the "play" as real as possible, because they know the important role that fear of the unknown plays in lowering a patient's threshold of pain. We observe examples of these effects of fear daily in the comparative freedom from pain that women delivering their second or third child have when contrasted with those experiencing childbirth for the first time.

On the day of the real operation, our patient was brought into the operating room at seven-fifteen in the morning. Hypnosis was induced forty minutes later, and within a few minutes catalepsy of the right arm indicated that a medium stage of hypnosis had been reached. The woman was completely alert but obviously much more at ease than patients about to receive a chemical anesthetic. After a while, the depth of her hypnotic state was deepened by repeated suggestions to breathe slower, deeper, and more regularly. She was told, too, that she was falling into a deep, sound, sleeplike state, and that the area of the incision was getting numb and insensitive to pain.

By eight-fifteen we were ready to begin the operation. The patient gave us only one sign that the affair was anything different from the "trial run" we had conducted a few weeks earlier. This was a mild complaint of pain at the time the towel clips were placed on her abdomen just before the skin incision was made. (Only then did we realize that this minor detail was inadvertently left out of the rehearsal.) Aside from that, however, there were no changes in her relaxed facial expression; nor were there any pain reflexes when the scalpel was used.

The woman conversed with her attendants during the entire operation. Her breathing continued to be slow, deep, and regular, and she stated that she felt no pain or discomfort. Clinically speaking, there was a gradual increase in the pulse rate during the extraction of the infant by forceps, which was complicated by the protrusion of the infant's shoulder and arm through the uterine incision. But when she observed the baby as it was delivered from her abdomen, our patient was ecstatic.

The total hysterectomy was begun at nine o'clock and completed at nine-forty. During this portion of the operation, the pulse rate dropped to slightly below normal levels, but the patient remained free of any sign of shock. When the operation was finally completed, she was given the post-hypnotic suggestion that she would have no postoperative pain, insomnia, or loss of appetite. She left the operating room in excellent condition; her postoperative course was uneventful; and she left the hospital on the tenth day following surgery.

From the physician's point of view, such good hypnotic subjects, who are comparatively rare, are a real pleasure to attend. But this is no less true in the larger number of instances in which the woman cannot "go all the way" with hypnosis and some form of chemoanesthesia is used in conjunction with suggestion. Sometimes these patients, especially those who have had operations on the upper part of the abdomen, are afraid to cough for fear of causing themselves pain. But simply by reinducing hypnosis, we can regulate this type of reaction.

You will need no help in interpreting the advantages of hypnosis in childbirth. They will be as apparent to you as they were to Mrs. S.O., a young mother whose memory of the normal, free-from-pain birth of her child is typical of hundreds of others on record. "When the time came to enter the hospital," she says, "I felt gay and relaxed—more like a person going to a special event than one preparing for delivery.

"There was no pain. I could feel the contractions. One would start at the base of my spine and spread across my abdomen. It would grow in intensity and then suddenly disappear. They were similar to bowel contractions, but stronger.

"When I was wheeled into the delivery room, I could not believe that I was actually ready. I kept expecting the doctor to send me home. The contractions were more frequent and stronger now, but still there was no pain. Between contractions, my body would go completely limp and relaxed. I thought about my husband out in the waiting room and hoped that he knew I was all right.

"The nurse seemed to be getting anxious. She kept asking if she should send for the anesthetist and warned: 'If you don't send for her now, it will be too late.' But the doctor said that in about three more pushes the baby would come. I didn't feel as though anything would happen in three more contractions that would require my receiving drugs. I had come this far: I was not going to weaken in the last few minutes.

"When the time for the last push came, the doctor said: 'Close your eyes. You are drifting off into a deep state of relaxation. When I say open your eyes, you will open them quickly and see your baby born. Now close your eyes.'

"I felt completely relaxed and contented. I had the feeling that I had floated peacefully right off the table. When the doctor asked if I could feel anything, I was feeling so lazy and content that I just didn't want to make the effort to answer. He repeated it twice, and I roused myself enough to say 'no.' He told me to push very hard, and as I did I felt a quick rotating downward movement. The doctor said, 'Open your eyes.' There was my baby crying and wiggling.

"How did it really feel to have my baby with hypnosis?

"It's not that frightening, hectic experience that some women expect. Everything seems very matter of fact. One event follows another in a routine fashion. All about you, people seem rushed and anxious, but you feel completely at ease. You are in such a state of mind that nothing could possibly upset you. You just lie there and wait—composed and patient.

"Afterwards, of course, it is thrilling to remember all the details and recall the joy and tenderness of that moment in your child's birth when you first laid eyes on him."

Hypnoanesthesia does, indeed, help make childbirth a most inviting experience. The reader must not permit herself to be dissuaded from the therapeutic applications of hypnosis in childbirth because we do not clearly understand just how hypnosis works. After all, we use electricity and do not know all about that either. The plain fact is that we do not know, for certain, *why* hypnosis relieves pain; nor do we, at present, understand the very nature of pain. However, we do know that the less-oriented woman is apt to experience more pain during the early phases of her labor than the well-prepared woman.

A second and more intense pain can arise in the dilating phase of delivery, especially if the woman is emotionally and intellectually unprepared for what is happening. This is the time when the excessive use of drugs for the relief of pain is particularly inadvisable, because the drugs do tend to retard labor. Depending upon a number of factors, the intermittent pains of the contracting uterus during this period can last for anywhere from six to ten hours, if unchecked.

Finally, there is the pain associated with the expulsion of the baby. Prior to the acceptance of hypnosis as a valuable ally in obstetrics by the medical profession, it was almost a universal practice to anesthetize patients at this stage of delivery. It was, therefore, a rare woman who knew the psychological uplift of witnessing the birth of her child. Of course, recent developments in childbirth "anesthesia" —such as spinal, saddle block, and novocain injections— enable every mother-to-be to witness the birth of her infant. However, here, too, hypnosis can decrease the fears, anxieties, and tensions that cannot be blocked off with any type of chemoanesthesia.

As explained in Chapter VI, we know that all pains, including those commonly associated with childbirth, travel along definitely traceable pathways of the body's nervous system. We know, too, that once such pains convey their messages to the brain—for example, alerting us to the fact that labor has begun—we have no further use for them. Considerable research on where the "blocking" of these pains occurs with hypnosis indicates that it takes place along those nerve highways to the brain.

The nerve fibers themselves are made up of many individual "wires," which are not continuous. Rather, they are loosely connected with each other at various switchlike junctures called "synapses." Just as an electric current is cut off at an open switch, stimulating impulses can be broken at these junction points along the nerve network. The most likely theory is that, in some still unexplained manner, the blocking of the pain transmission takes place in this area with hypnoanesthesia.

We could go on to probe other "whys" of the nervous

system and brain, and our efforts would take us into fascinating corners of the mind. In each of us, for instance, the impulses that we receive are stored in "memory cells" located in the brain. We each have some ten to fifteen billion of these cells with a capacity to store about one hundred thousand memories apiece. These cells form the center of recall for all painful as well as pleasurable experiences. During an average life span, this memory bank can contain over seventy trillion separate bits of information, such as the fact that a hot stove burns. It is vital to our comfort and safety that we retain memories of this type. But, in most instances, no value can be attached to recalling the pains of childbirth. With hypnoanesthesia, we choose the memories we wish to retain.

The reader interested in delving further into the physiology of pain can find a great deal more on this subject in her physician's library. At the moment, we know that you are more concerned with the results rather than with the methodology of pain-relieving measures. In fact, without knowing why they work, you have probably been using the principles of suggestion since your own childhood days. The "dry run" visit to the hospital a day or two before you went to have your tonsils removed and the kiss your mother bestowed upon your hurt finger made these experiences less painful, even though you could not explain why.

In adult life, too, all of us function in much the same manner. We have an interesting example of this in a very recent study by Dr. John B. Ross of the reactions of twelve thousand blood donors as reported to the American Association of Blood Banks. Dr. Ross states that the fainting of some adults when they are called upon to give blood appears to be a psychosomatic phenomenon. It is a form of escape, he says, from what the donor imagines to be an unpleasant task.

Does this sound familiar? It should. And so should this: Dr. Ross goes on to explain that the body responds to this below-conscious desire to flee by diverting blood to the muscles from other parts of the body—particularly the brain. This, plus the fact that social circumstances do not permit the person to run from donating his blood, leaves him with just one escape—fainting. Practically all doctors connected with this noble work observe that, in contrast, the professional donor who gives blood for a fee is more relaxed because of repeated experiences.

As for the "kissing" trick your mother used so effectively— you can observe phenomena like this for yourself almost any day. The next time you are hurt and you have done everything possible to make yourself physically comfortable, try closing your eyes and doing your very best to recall everything that happened just before the pain struck. Was someone else present in the room? If so, what was he or she saying? What were you doing? How was the room decorated? Most important, what were your emotions? Were you happy, sad, or, perhaps, fearful? If you will repeat these attempts at recall six or seven times, or often enough so that everything connected with the painful event is vividly clear, you will realize that nothing preceding that event was necessarily painful. You will see the pain in its proper perspective—as the result of an isolated event that is certainly not repeating itself. Shorn of any exaggerated importance you might have attached to it, the pain should either diminish or disappear completely.

When we are young and unable to figure such things out for ourselves, we can accomplish the same thing by concentrating our awareness on a handy distraction—mother's kiss. "Hypnosis!" you say. Well, is that not what we are talking about?

Before we leave the subject of hypnosis and pain, particularly as it relates to childbirth, we should emphasize that no two subjects will ever react exactly the same to hypnoanesthesia. You may be able to control pain with nothing more than light hypnosis; your neighbor may require deep somnambulism to achieve the same results; and still another woman may not be able to respond to suggestion at all. Furthermore, pain is not an absolute factor in our lives. At a certain moment of a particular day, the slightest discomfort may loom large in your mind as an "unbearable" pain. The very next moment, you might hardly notice it at all, because the influences on your threshold of pain are vast and complicated.

For these reasons, chemical anesthesia is always available in a delivery room, even when the patient is an excellent hypnotic subject. There is never any thought of making childbirth an endurance contest for the mother by "shaming" her into going through the experience with hypnosis alone. As a matter of record, chemoanesthesia is used in conjunction with hypnosis in all but less than ten per cent of our patients. You should, therefore, know what some of these chemicals are and what you may expect of them. However, the decision to use any one or a combination of them will rest squarely with your obstetrician. He is trained to protect not only your comfort but also your health.

Very likely you have heard of the spinal or continuous caudal anesthesia that we mentioned earlier. For a while, after its introduction into the field of obstetrics eighteen years ago, it was widely acclaimed as the "perfect" anesthetic for childbirth, because it leaves the mother completely conscious while insuring that the pains of her labors do not get through to the reception centers of her brain.

The method employed here is to inject a drug into the spinal canal or into the nerves as they emerge just outside of it, at a point a little lower on the body at the extreme end of the vertebral column. The object of this injection is to deaden the sensations of the nerves that carry pain impulses up through the spinal column to the brain. With its multitude of entwined nerves, this column is the Los Angeles Freeway of the nervous system's highway network. Pain at this point is blocked by the numbing solution, which saturates all of the nerves in the column. Unfortunately, the effect lasts for a short while only and the anesthetic must be repeatedly renewed if the relief is to be extended for several hours.

Another chemical anesthetic that, for a while, was more popular with patients and physicians than it is today is known as "twilight sleep." Actually, this is a combination of two drugs—morphine and scopolamine. Rather than being a pain-relieving agent, the latter is more of a memory-suppressing drug. Thus, while the morphine does alleviate some of the pain, the woman still experiences most of the discomforts of childbirth with twilight sleep. Yet, afterwards, thanks to the scopolamine, she does not remember any of the pain and suffering that she might have gone through. It is easy to see how such a drug could win popular approval as fast as this one did early in the century. But time has taught us to respect the detrimental effect that it can have upon the ability of the baby to breathe at birth.

The other half of twilight sleep, morphine, has consistently been one of the most widely-used drugs in alleviating the pains occurring during childbirth. It is easily administered by hypodermic needle, and it does, in fact, "take the edge off" pain in the dilating stage of labor for an hour or so. However, unless the drug is judiciously administered, this respite for the mother can be won at the risk of inhibiting labor or, worse yet, introducing the harmful effects of the morphine into the blood stream of the infant.

Interestingly, it was hypnosis (or rather the absence of it) which led to the professional discovery of still another chemical anesthetic—nitrous oxide, popularly known as "laughing gas." On the night of December 10, 1844, a dentist named Horace Wells was in the audience of a Hartford, Connecticut, theater. While a professional magician on stage was presumably demonstrating hypnosis, his assistant in the wings was actually engulfing the subjects in the gas. Wells observed that one of these subjects accidentally fell and struck his leg against a chair without experiencing any pain. At that moment the dentist conceived the dream of painless dentistry based upon the use of nitrous oxide, and the gas was on its way to becoming a respectable tool of the healing professions.

Today we use nitrous oxide extensively in childbirth, especially in the final stages of delivery. The routine is, usually, to give the patient a few whiffs of the gas, upon request, at the beginning of a contraction. This is generally sufficient to dull the pain without inhibiting the labor. In fact, the woman, under the influence of those few deep breaths of the gas, may carry out the procedure of "bearing down" without being consciously aware of it. She awakens between contractions, and the entire procedure is repeated. Finally, as the moment of birth nears, the quantity of anesthetic administered is increased so that the mother is actually unconscious at the climax of her efforts.

We could go on to list numerous other chemical anesthetics, such as paraldehyde, rectal ether, and all the different barbiturates. Each has an advantage which might prove helpful in your delivery, and your physician can certainly advise you in your choice. But you can help yourself by remembering that these valuable discoveries are most effective when used as an ally—never as a crutch.

CHAPTER VIII

•

Other Hypnotic Phenomena

HYPNOSIS, OR SUGGESTION, has many other uses besides controlling pain. Fortunately, most of these "plus" benefits do not require the depth of hypnosis indicated for hypnoanesthesia, and so they are within the reach of almost all persons, whether or not they are easily hypnotizable. Long after your baby is born, for example, you still may be employing the principles you have learned in order either to relax or to sleep more soundly. You can also cure yourself of a distasteful habit, recall an important fact temporarily lost in that crowded memory bank of yours, or, conversely, forget some searing experience that you just cannot seem to put out of your mind in any other way. These are merely a few of the conscious uses you can make of the procedures and practices we have been discussing. Actually, the complete list of the applications of suggestion encompasses every act you perform, whether it is consciously thought out or not—even just helping you to decide which brand of toothpaste you will buy.

Closer to home for us, in the fields of medicine, hypnosis has come of age in still other directions. It is being recommended by doctors in increasing numbers as part of the therapy for a great many illnesses other than the psychosomatically-based allergies. With sometimes astoundingly swift results, it has already been used in the treatment of disturbing dreams and nightmares, especially among younger patients; hypochondria; nervous habits; fears and anxieties; depressions; and a host of other neurotic disturbances. It is employed more and more, too, as part of the over-all treatment for drug addiction and alcoholism. Finally, of course, suggestion is undeniably influential in both causing and alleviating many of the discomforts of pregnancy.

We shall have more to say about how hypnosis can help you to handle these specific discomforts in Chapter IX. Before we get to this, however, let us take a closer look at some of the other phenomena of hypnosis, beginning with those which exert the greatest influence on our daily lives. After all, childbirth with hypnosis is simply an extension of these same familiar influences, just as surely as childbirth itself is an extension of life.

Suppose we start with a most common bedtime scene. It is the end of an extremely hectic day. You are very tired, and you feel as if you could sleep clear through the next twenty-four hours. But you have an important appointment early in the morning, so, just before you fall asleep, you "set" your mind to awaken at a certain hour. Perhaps you even imagine the hands of the clock as they will appear at the exact moment in the morning when you want to open your eyes. If you are like many people, you will be able to do this easily. Furthermore, if you tell yourself at night that you will not only awaken on time but that you will also feel rested and refreshed, the chances are excellent that you will arrive promptly for your appointment feeling both alert and relaxed.

Probably you already recognize the fact that this business of awakening at a predetermined hour is a common, everyday example of what we have been calling "posthypnotic suggestion." We say "*post*hypnotic," because these suggestions are effective after the suggestions we give ourselves to fall asleep. As a subject, you will encounter this interesting phenomenon of hypnosis formally from your very first session when, just before he alerts you, your doctor suggests that, in subsequent sessions, you will be speedily hypnotized when he gives you some simple signal. This is a valuable timesaving device, and it helps to nullify the complaint of some physicians that hypnosis is too lengthy a procedure to be of practical value. After an initial indoctrination session, you can go into a deep hypnotic state at any time within a matter of seconds, if you are a good subject. The signal for this deep relaxation, which must be agreed upon beforehand by both you and your doctor, might be anything from a word or a gesture to a light touch on, perhaps, the shoulder.

There are, of course, many other uses for posthypnotic suggestions besides rehypnotizing subjects. One of the more important of these is the speedier healing of wounds. Postoperative patients who are not prepared hypnotically to experience less pain usually require larger doses of narcotics for relief. The narcotics, in turn, inhibit the patients' appetites, and the resulting poor nutrition retards the wound-healing, prolonging the suffering in what can be a vicious cycle.

Other areas where posthypnotic suggestion is effective are to be seen in cases where patients must adjust to the wearing of certain uncomfortable medical or dental appliances. Except in those cases of abnormal fear of injection, the use of chemoanesthesia in the dentist's office is usually sufficient to alleviate any pain that might occur. On the other hand, there is no chemical that will completely eliminate the discomfort to the wearer of a new set of dentures or that will inhibit the gagging reflex common to such a patient. To control this tendency in a subject capable of reaching a deep state of hypnosis, a dentist may merely suggest: "In the future, you will not gag. Fifteen times a day, you will lick your lips when you feel like gagging, but you will not gag." The effect of this suggestion, after several weekly visits during which hypnosis is induced and that posthypnotic suggestion is made, is to replace the distressing habit of gagging with the more comfortable one of lip-licking, so that the patient soon requires no further therapy.

We could go on to list a hundred or more common complaints that can be treated with posthypnotic suggestion. These would include many illnesses which, at first glance, might seem to fall more within the realm of the psychoanalyst than that of the hypnotically-oriented physician. All of the psychosomatic ailments or detrimental habits—such as smoking, drinking, and overeating—would be good examples. Now we do not intend to debate the relative merits of psychoanalysis and hypnotherapy. Each of these undoubtedly has its place in the medical armamentarium. Yet, as efficient as analysis might be in some cases, it is still an involved, lengthy technique that must be ruled out when time is a factor—as in the case of childbirth. In addition, we cannot be positive that psychoanalysis, which carefully screens the patients it finally does accept, will provide permanent relief from emotionally-based discomforts.

Quite frankly, this latter objection applies to hypnotherapy, too. Posthypnotic suggestions may last for minutes or years, but they do not last forever. They must be continually reinforced by additional suggestions for as long as it takes the patient to develop a better behavior pattern and to eliminate the need for further implantation of the suggestion. Just how long posthypnotic suggestions remain effective depends upon a number of factors. First and foremost of these is the attitude of the subject—you. If the suggestion is contrary to your true wishes, it will have no greater posthypnotic effect than it would have had while you were hypnotized—which is to say, for all practical purposes, no effect at all. Second, the nature of the suggestion and the manner in which it is phrased will bear heavily upon how long after hypnosis the suggestion will continue to have some influence upon your behavior.

Third—and this is possibly most important of all—those very principles of confidence and expectancy which we mentioned earlier will determine how long a posthypnotic suggestion will remain effective. You are positively in full control of the situation. If you believe that you will respond or behave in a certain manner moments or months from now, the chances are excellent that you will.

Naturally, in obstetrical cases, where we are primarily concerned with the patient's comfort for a few months, we usually do not have to worry about posthypnotic suggestions' losing their effect. Between regular office visits and home practice in autohypnosis, you will have ample opportunity to reinforce such suggestions as: "I will happily look forward to having my baby. I will have no fear and will feel no pain or discomfort." Merely by following a few simple rules and suggestions, you can keep such thoughts uppermost in your mind until after your baby is born.

All of this, of course, is to give you some background in the very nature of posthypnotic suggestion. *After* your baby is born, you will find countless practical uses for posthypnotic suggestions, which you may give yourself via autohypnosis or which your physician may want to give you while you are deeply relaxed. These applications of posthypnotic suggestion during your postnatal period will include many things from the relief of many types of constipation to improving your memory. The actual list embraces literally hundreds of other medical and nonmedical uses but, as is the case with hypnosis, it is best to consult your physician before attempting to alleviate any discomfort yourself with posthypnotic suggestion.

Our primary concern here, however, is with the use of

hypnotic phenomena in childbirth. Let us consider another one of these, which has, in certain selected cases, proved beneficial to patients. With these women—and we cannot emphasize too strongly that the selection must be made by the physician—we have actually initiated labor several weeks before the baby was due. All of these women were, of course, good or somnambulistic subjects who were already mothers. The memories of this earlier experience with childbirth were never removed from the patients' memory banks and, thus, could be reactivated.

One of these patients, Mrs. J.R., twenty-seven years old, was several weeks from term when she was examined by several reputable obstetricians who doubted very much that labor could be induced by even chemical means. Nevertheless, with the patient's permission, she was hypnotized and brought back (regressed) to the time of her previous delivery—three and a half years earlier. We mean, of course, that the patient was asked to call upon the memories of that particular experience. We did not give her the suggestion that she would go into labor. Rather, we suggested that she would actually re-experience all of the subjective sensations that she had had during the initial stages of that previous labor. For example, she was told that she would vividly recall being shaved and given an enema, that she would remember the exact manner in which her contractions began, and that she would recall the ache in the back spreading around to the abdomen.

As a result of these efforts and the patient's complete co-operation, within twenty minutes after the suggestions were given, and while the patient was still under deep hypnosis, the contractions of her uterus were readily discernible. These became progressively stronger until, a little more than six hours later, she delivered a healthy infant.

CHILDBIRTH WITH HYPNOSIS

We have observed other similar cases of hypnotically-induced labor. However, all of these have been with the second, or some other subsequent, pregnancy. Although the use of hypnosis for the induction of labor with women in their first pregnancy has been recorded, we seriously doubt that this can be done. There is, after all, no experience on deposit in the memory bank upon which these women can draw.

The study of age regression and its still more vivid form, revivification, can take us far afield from our purpose here. But one incident involving the supposed use of these hypnotic phenomena is worth mentioning, because it forms the basis for so much misunderstanding about hypnosis today.

Not so many years ago (in 1952), an incident that occurred in Pueblo, Colorado, focused world attention on hypnosis, generally, and age regression and revivification, specifically. A well-informed, amateur hypnotist, Morey Bernstein, succeeded in inducing a deep somnambulistic state of hypnosis in a twenty-nine-year-old housewife.

While his subject was in this extremely relaxed frame of mind—and with her explicit permission—Bernstein requested that she recall certain events out of her past. His account of this experiment, published as a best-selling book, *The Search for Bridey Murphy*, purported to show that this twentieth-century American woman could remember not only events as far back as her infancy but also those things which, supposedly, took place in an "earlier life" as Bridey Murphy—a nineteenth-century Irish housewife.

Any discussion of Bernstein's work quite obviously tends to lure one into adopting a stand either for or against believing in reincarnation. We shall try to avoid that pitfall. As for the balance of his experiment—we do not believe that any individual can be brought back even to the first few months of his *present* existence with hypnosis.

The "Bridey Murphy" incident was a case of both the investigator's and his subject's being taken in by still another aspect of hypnosis: that is that even in the deepest hypnotic state, the subject does not cease to use her imagination. It is probable that Bernstein's subject, having been subjected to *accounts* of life as an Irish housewife sometime in her consciously-forgotten past, was able to recall these stories with hypnosis. Such incidents are often expressed as very real events by highly-imaginative subjects, so that only a skilled physician is able to distinguish between fact and fiction.

When we speak of "age regression" in hypnosis, we are referring to the ability of a subject to recall certain events which took place during an earlier period of her life. Again, depending upon many variables, not the least important of which is the depth of the hypnotic stage reached, this ability can span a period ranging from just "yesterday" to the subject's earliest childhood. All of these events, however, appear in the light of, and in relation to, the knowledge and attitudes acquired by the subject since their original occurrence. For example, with hypnosis you may regress to a certain day in grade school when the boy behind you pulled your pigtails; but in recalling that event as an adult, it will seem far less tragic than it did when it happened.

Somnambulism is a prime requisite to any regression. The doctor relaxes his subject to the point where she does not know, or even care to know, the period of time in which she is now living. Beyond that, the technique is based upon that same rapport between subject and operator which must exist in order for all hypnotic phenomena to be effective. Dr. Louis R. Wolberg, whose research in the field of hypnoanalysis is well known both in this country and abroad, and who could hardly be accused of taking anything less than a scientific approach towards his subject, has formulated an interesting method of inducing regression.

"Now concentrate carefully upon what I have to say," he tells a deeply-hypnotized patient. "I am going to suggest that you go back into the past. You will feel as if you were back in the period I suggest.

"Let us start with yesterday. What did you do yesterday morning? What did you have for breakfast? For lunch? Now we are going back to the first day you came to see me. Can you *see* yourself talking to me? How did you feel? Describe it. What clothes did you wear?

"Now listen carefully. We are going back to a period when you were little. You are getting smaller. . . . You are getting smaller and smaller. . . . Your arms and legs are getting smaller. I am someone you know and like. You are between ten and twelve years old. Can you see yourself?

"Describe what you see. . . . Now you are getting even smaller. You are becoming very, very little. Your arms and legs are shrinking. Your body is shrinking. . . . You are going back to a time when you were very, very little. . . . Now you are a very little child. You are going back to the time when you entered school for the first time.

"Can you see yourself? Who is your teacher? How old are you? What are your friends' names? Now you are even smaller than that. You are very, very much smaller. Your mother is holding you. Do you see yourself with your mother? What is she wearing? What is she saying?"

With procedures such as the one just described, we are able to regress co-operative patients to their very earliest years. There is, at present, no proof available that anyone has ever been regressed to a prenatal level. But it is fairly common for hypnotically-oriented physicians to regress to the grade-school period patients who are thirty or forty years old. During these sessions, the patient may speak, write, and even think as she did during those long-ago moments. And there have been fewer, but no less amazing, instances of regressing subjects to the preschool level so that they are unable to write or even speak, because they had not mastered the forms of communication at that stage of life. Instead, they exhibit the thumb-sucking and grasping movements of the infant. As we have already indicated, when the subject actually relives, rather than merely recalls, those early stages of her development, without regard or relation to subsequently-acquired knowledge or attitudes, the phenomenon is known as "revivification."

There seems to be no doubt that good subjects can "think themselves back" as far as their childhood. And there is also no doubt that they can return, none the worse for the journey back through time, and resume their normal adult behavior patterns immediately upon being alerted. Furthermore, as we noted earlier in this chapter, regression or revivification, in the hands of a skilled physician, can do a great deal of good for the patient.

It is interesting to observe, too, that there are several valid scientific tests for detecting the subject who "pretends" to be regressed because she wants to be considered a good sport, or because she desires to be the center of attention, or because of some other reason. One of these is the test for the "Babinski" reflex. You can observe this reflex action for yourself by lightly running your finger along the bottom of a baby's foot. You will note that his big toe will curl upward and that the other toes will tend to spread apart. This peculiar reaction is common to only the youngest infants. It usually vanishes before the children begin to walk or talk. However, some subjects who know nothing at all about this response have demonstrated it under hypnotic revivification, thereby establishing the validity of their voyage back through time. A patient who is pretending, unless she knows of the response, will obviously not demonstrate it.

It is all too easy to imagine the lengths to which we can go with age regression or revivification. Just as warm, pleasant moments out of the distant past may be recalled, long-forgotten incidents or fears that have left psychological scars on our personalities may be exposed for treatment with modern therapeutic techniques. In fact, these hypnotic phenomena have contributed greatly to our understanding of *why* the Freudian psychoanalytic method works. The important thing to remember, particularly as a subject, is that there is nothing mysterious or frightening about the induction of regressive states. Perhaps because this induction is a bit more difficult to comprehend than is, say, posthypnotic suggestion, it has been the object of much rumor and half-truth. Actually, it may be compared with simpler memory recall through concentration of awareness. With regression or revivification, the memory simply becomes so real that the subject seems to relive events gone by. If you have ever been "carried away" by a daydream, you will readily understand how easy it is to become "lost" in a memory in this manner.

Before your baby is born, you will probably have little use for regression. The time required to induce the depth of hypnosis necessary for this phenomenon precludes its use in handling most of the fears and anxieties encountered in normal pregnancies. Also, these fears can be adequately controlled with other, simpler techniques. Yet your physician may suggest this procedure to expose the source of your faulty attitudes towards childbirth or your other psychological blocks to a happy, comfortable delivery. After childbirth, though, you will have even more of an opportunity to work with your physician to apply the techniques that we have been discussing towards achieving a fuller, richer life.

Although we sometimes see remarkable personality changes—usually for the better—in women who have just become mothers, you should not *expect* childbirth to make you more secure, more mature in your outlook, or more pleasant to live with than you were before. Such facets of your personality have been a lifetime in developing. They are the product of certain inherited physical characteristics plus literally thousands of impressive experiences. The vast majority of these impressions lie buried deep in your subconscious mind. Normally, you do not know that they are there. (We have already noted how this experiential background can produce pain and other physical symptoms of distress.) And prior to the present, widely-accepted state of hypnosis, about the only method that a patient had to root out these particularly disturbing experiences was to submit to psychoanalysis or some other form of extreme psychotherapy.

That, at any rate, was what Mrs. G.N., a young mother who complained of a severe pain in the lower part of her back following the delivery of her child, would have had to do. This patient had a rapid and painless two-and-one-half-hour labor with a comparatively mild chemical anesthetic. She delivered a perfectly healthy, beautiful child. By all indications, her postnatal period should have been uneventful. But throughout her confinement she complained of the backache, which became so severe that ten days later she could not leave the hospital. Instead of responding to all the usual forms of treatment, the pains had spread to her left leg.

The constant, unrelieved pain, as well as negative indications on a battery of tests which we performed at the hospital, made us think that perhaps we were dealing with a psychosomatic manifestation rather than a purely physical problem. Because the patient was very intelligent and readily gave her permission, we tried to relieve her distress with hypnosis.

The first few sessions were spent in conditioning her to the procedure we would follow, because she was, up until that moment, unfamiliar with hypnotic routine. It was not long, however, before the patient could reach a deep, somnambulistic state of relaxation, and in that state she could move about freely without any sign of pain. Furthermore, while hypnotized, she revealed that she had expected to have "pains of labor" and that because her labor had been free of pain, she felt that she had "missed something."

Several sessions later, while in the relaxed, free-talking state of hypnosis, she stated that her backache recurred whenever she saw her mother-in-law, with whom she and her husband had been living. She said, too, that she did not want to have her baby and that her sexual relations with her husband, whom she truly loved, were far from satisfactory. "Even though he is very considerate, I wish he would be more firm and masculine!" she exclaimed. These things and more were revealed at the same time to both the patient and her physician. The reaction of the patient, in itself, was exceedingly interesting. "Perhaps," she mused, "if *I* probe a little deeper, I will find the reason for my backache."

While getting this patient to regress to the period preceding her pregnancy, it was established that she had had a strong emotional attachment for the gentleman for whom she had worked at the time. "My old boss," she said, "was handsome, ambitious, meticulous, and just perfect in every way." When our patient was two months pregnant, this man, whom she so admired, died. "I wanted to name my baby after him, and my husband objected and became very angry," she recalled.

Following these most revealing periods, the patient was advised to leave her mother-in-law's home and to establish a home of her own with her husband and child. With the aid of deep hypnosis, she came to the realization that she was not in love with her husband but was actually in love with her dead employer. It was apparent to her that her backache was an alibi for her present unhappy marital status. She saw, also, that it was foolish to be in love with a dead man, and she decided that a more healthy attitude towards her husband was possible—as indeed it was.

Boiled down to its essentials for the purpose of discussion here, this case, which was successfully terminated within several months after the first complaint, illustrates a modern, widely-accepted form of therapy called "hypnoanalysis." With this procedure, treatment of many emotional disorders, at the hands of a qualified medical person, is possible. Depending upon the individual circumstances, any one or all of the hypnotic phenomena may be used. The technique enables the patient to understand the reasons for her reactions and enables her to come to grips with the causative factors responsible for her symptoms.

At no time is the patient subservient, unconscious, or helpless. Rather, she gains insight into her problem by reliving old behavior patterns through the use of regressive-like phenomena. She then understands the origin and the basis of her symptoms, and she discovers for herself how they are linked with life's experiences, childhood pattern formations, and faulty patterns of thinking.

When the meaning of these faulty attitudes becomes clear *to the patient*, the symptoms themselves will disappear. Contrary to the opinion held by some Freudian psychoanalysts, with hypnoanalysis there is never any direct suggestion to the patient that "you will get well." Nor do we indulge in mere "symptom removal" with posthypnotic suggestion or some other temporary cure. Relief from the distressing neurotic symptoms is obtained because the patient understands the emotional need for getting sick in the first place.

You should not make the mistake of supposing, however, that you must be "sick" in order to benefit from such phenomena as age regression and posthypnotic suggestion. In addition to hypnoanalysis, the uses of regression, for example, include a better understanding of why our family and friends behave towards us as they do. What is to us an inconsequential remark made long ago and forgotten may have aggravated another person all those years. And it is just this type of experience that can lead to some of the otherwise unexplainable aches and pains of which many women complain during pregnancy.

As for posthypnotic suggestion—the most common, though far from only, use by serious students of hypnosis is to break distasteful habits. In the following chapters, we shall relate several of these habits (e.g., overeating) to the discomforts of pregnancy and we shall show how simply but effectively they may be broken. However, for the present, let us imagine that, during or after your pregnancy, you decide to break the cigarette-smoking habit.

You may do this either by following the posthypnotic suggestions of your hypnotist or, under the guidance of your physician, by using autohypnosis. In either case, after you have reached a fairly deep state of hypnosis, you will light a cigarette. Your doctor will say: "As you take deep puffs on the cigarette, you will notice that the first puff will be slightly bitter. . . . There, you can detect that bitter taste now. You don't like it at all. When you take your second, third, and fourth puffs, that taste will grow even more bitter. It will be very distasteful—so distasteful that you'll positively hate it. You'll crush the cigarette out."

If you persist in smoking after the first few suggestions of bitterness, you will finally reach a point where the taste is so disagreeable that you will throw the cigarette away after the very first puff. How long that will take is strictly a matter between yourself and your imagination. When it finally does occur, you will be given the posthypnotic suggestion that even after you are alerted, you will continue to taste that same bitterness every time you smoke. "You'll get to dislike smoking," your therapist will suggest, "and you'll smoke fewer and fewer cigarettes."

There is, of course, no guarantee that you can break the cigarette-smoking habit with hypnosis alone. As we have said, posthypnotic suggestions must be renewed from time to time. Also, you must be capable of achieving an effective depth of hypnosis in order for posthypnotic suggestions to work. Within these limits, though, and with the aid of auto-hypnosis, you can break the cigarette-smoking habit, or any other habit for that matter, if you can imagine yourself doing it and if you really want to stop.

CHAPTER IX

•

Discomforts of
Pregnancy

FROM THE VERY conception of the child, the birth process is one vast emotional experience, which is truly magnificent for some women, disturbing for others, and downright frightening for still others. Which type it will be for you depends, to a large extent, upon your background, training, and outlook. Fortunately, if you are in a class with the great majority of women, you will be a happy, contented obstetric patient, refusing to believe that the birth of your child can be anything but a joyous, deeply-satisfying peak to your role as a woman in this world. Investigations of this attitude in many of our patients reveal that it is based upon a healthy emotional development during the formative years of the mother-to-be. An adequate sex education, a well-handled adolescent period, a satisfactory and normal marital adjustment, and, of course, a genuine desire for the child also play constructive parts in the drama.

However, childbirth may just as easily loom as a frightening, painful specter against the wrong psychosexual background. If pregnancy occurs before a woman has completely adjusted to her marriage, or if the husband reacts unfavorably towards the pregnancy, the wife's attitude towards her own condition will be adversely affected. Some of the other causes for this "rejection" of pregnancy may be economic problems, the number of children already in the family, and the fear that marital relations will suffer by the child's coming between the parents.

For some women, the physical and social limitations imposed by the pregnancy are sufficient cause for the resentment and rejection of it. Others, knowingly or not, may not wish to bear a child because they imagine that it will interfere with a career. Occasionally, especially in those instances where the husband and relatives pamper the wife and make a "baby" out of her, the woman's neurotic satisfactions may be increased. But she will then reject the child as a competitor for this attention.

When many immature, dependent females, whose mothers always did everything for them, are faced with labor, they wish that their mothers could have their babies for them. For such women, labor may be a difficult, emotional experience characterized by tumultuous contractions of the uterus. As a result, excessive drugging is necessary to reduce the intensity of the discomfort. Training in hypnosis, in order to give these patients a sense of self-esteem and self-reliance, has been particularly successful.

It is true that many of those women who do not desire pregnancy for one reason or another do resign themselves to it with apparent fairly good grace when it does occur. For a small number, however, some form of deep and adequate psychotherapy may be required. In any event, we are certain that women who do not want children are usually psychosexually immature and generally reject to some degree the feminine role.

Sometimes even the desire *for* a child can have unhealthy psychological overtones. We frequently encounter women who view their pregnancies as a means of getting support, inheritance, or holding indifferent husbands. There are many classical instances of mothers who desire children for the purpose of vicariously reliving their own unsatisfactory lives. The so-called "stage mother" is a typical example of this latter type.

Finally, some women use their pregnant states as a lever for demanding more of their husbands' attention and love, because they now fear the loss of this love as a result of the distortion of their figures. Naturally, when these are the primary reasons for wanting a child, the maneuvers inevitably fail and the cycle of emotional disturbances is further accelerated.

The very first indications of neurotic problems that can interfere with the smooth course of birth in an otherwise healthy married woman may be signs of frigidity or sexual coldness or the development of a complete aversion towards sexual contacts. It is not, however, absolutely essential to conception for the woman to reach a climax of pleasure in natural intercourse. In fact, Dr. Robert R. Knight reported in a Menninger Clinic bulletin, some ten years before the celebrated Kinsey Report was made public, that perhaps seventy-five per cent of all married women derive little or no pleasure from the sex act.

"Many not only experience no pleasure," he wrote, "but actually suffer revulsion and pain." Despite this far from satisfactory state of marital affairs, an overwhelming majority of these women go right on bearing children conceived with their husbands. The pity of it all is that having a baby for such women can be a hollow triumph. Instead of relieving their tensions, the patients displace these onto their offspring, thus perpetuating an endless procession of neurotic generations.

Nearly all of the women whom we see on this score present themselves to us, at first, with complaints of pelvic pain, excessive bleeding, backache, migraine headache, or any one of a host of other symptoms that serve merely as alibis for the lack of sexual gratification. Some of these patients have even had *two* abdominal operations without relief of the basic complaint.

Of course, surgery is valueless. A close inspection of the attitudes of these patients reveals an almost identical pattern of flight from reality and combat with the environment interwoven with the marriage thread. The marital union may be characterized by the refusal of the woman to assume any serious obligation of wifehood or motherhood. There is also generally an abnormal interest in card-playing or club and sports activities, with a proportionate neglect of the husband. This type of person will commonly take great interest in traveling alone, purchasing expensive clothes, or perhaps even the aggressive pursuit of a career. Always, pregnancy is avoided as a nuisance or even a calamity.

Nausea and vomiting

Perhaps you have heard that physicians sometimes refer to pregnancy as "a disease of nine-months duration." Unquestionably, the reason for this "hard-boiled" attitude of some doctors is the multitude of aches, pains, and complaints—all apparently unrelated to physical changes in pregnancy—that many patients seem to share. In early pregnancy, for example, nearly half of all women experience nausea and some vomiting. Severe vomiting, though, is much less frequent than some of the gossip concerning childbirth would lead us to suspect. Still, the numerous drugs on the market for controlling nausea in pregnancy indicate just how real that problem is. The variety of these chemicals is in itself proof that none of these remedies has proved exceptionally successful, except in isolated cases.

As discomforts of pregnancy, nausea and vomiting appear to be particularly prevalent in women of our own Western civilization. The incidence of this symptom is low among the Eskimo and native African tribes. It is only slightly more common with Negroes in the southern United States. Scientists have been attempting for many years to explain these variations on the basis of a difference in diet. It is more likely, however, that the lower incidence of nausea in certain groups is due to the phlegmatic personalities of the people. The stoic Oriental, for instance, is seldom known to have what her American sisters call "morning sickness." Both the placid American and Mexican Indians, too, are comparatively free from this discomfort. Yet when members of these groups become assimilated into our society, with its heightened tempo and attendant neurosis, morning sickness becomes one of the first signs of pregnancy.

Certainly we must not completely forget that there may be very real physical causes for nausea in pregnancy—or at any other time, for that matter. The symptom could indicate a stomach ulcer, tumor, or bowel and bladder disturbance, to mention just a few of the possibilities. Your physician will want to check for all of those before investigating still other possible causes.

However, the evidence in favor of this discomfort's being psychosomatic in origin is overwhelming. Aside from comparing the different reactions of various racial and national groups, we have noted that women who complain of premenstrual distress almost always have nausea and vomiting when they are pregnant. A study of our own patients with this complaint reveals that in practically every case the symptom is either an expression of unconscious rejection of the pregnancy or a misguided indicator that the woman gives herself to prove that she is really pregnant. This latter type of patient has been literally "brainwashed" by gossip into accepting the notion that "morning sickness" is a necessary beginning to all pregnancy.

The interesting point is that, except in very rare instances, the nausea and vomiting disappear by the fourth or fifth month of pregnancy—when the body has adjusted to the hormone imbalance caused by the pregnancy—even though no therapy is attempted. We strongly believe that, by that time, the mother-to-be, both consciously and unconsciously, has accepted the fact that she is pregnant. She also has begun to recognize that the fetus is a separate living being, not something to be ignored or "thrown up."

As early as 1946, the author, together with Dr. S. T. De-Lee, reported in the *American Journal of Obstetrics and Gynecology* how a series of refractory, or pernicious, vomiters was dramatically cured by hypnotherapy in anywhere from one visit to six visits. All of these patients were very sick: for many, therapeutic abortion was being considered as a lifesaving procedure.

One such patient, Mrs. E.H., twenty-five years old and expecting her third child, had been hospitalized twice before early in her pregnancy for severe nausea and vomiting. Less than two weeks after her release from the hospital, she was back for a third time. The symptoms were still the same, but now, after many futile attempts at purely medical treatment, her bodily condition was beginning to deteriorate further. Hypnosis was suggested as a last resort.

The patient was placed in a deep somnambulistic state. By means of direct as well as posthypnotic suggestion, it was emphasized that the vomiting would cease at once and that she would be able to eat and retain her meals. The completely relaxed woman was left in this deep state for two hours. When she was alerted, an obvious change in her condition was seen. Her fears, anxieties, and excitability were gone, and she stated that she "felt great." She began to eat again—small feedings at first, and then larger ones. She retained food, suffered no nausea, and continued to improve. Ten days later, she left the hospital to complete an otherwise uneventful prenatal course.

Hypnosis, in this instance, was instrumental in saving the

life of this woman's unborn child. While it is reassuring to know that such therapy is available, your own discomforts need never reach such serious proportions. It is quite probable that, if you apply the basic techniques of relaxation that you have learned and follow such common-sense advice as "stop talking while you're eating," you will experience a minimum amount of trouble. This is particularly worth remembering if you are inclined to be naturally tense, because the "nervous" and compulsive swallowing of air can be an important factor in producing nausea and vomiting.

As for those emotional problems—thanks to the efforts of many research-minded physicians, we are closer than ever before to knowing exactly how important they are at this particular stage of pregnancy. In 1957, Drs. Stephen W. Giorlando and Richard F. Mascola reported on their investigations of a dozen cases of hyperemesis gravidarum (severe nausea and vomiting in pregnancy) at the Lutheran Hospital in Brooklyn, New York. The results of this research, with particular emphasis on hypnotherapy as a form of treatment, have been summarized in the following highly-illuminating table:

Now what can you learn from these cold statistics? First of all, we should point out that the one case of spontaneous abortion (L.C.) had a history of similar difficulty. Her first pregnancy had terminated with a spontaneous abortion at eight weeks. Another patient (H.G.), however, who had aborted spontaneously in a first pregnancy, carried to full-term this time and gave birth to a healthy son. What is more important, we believe, is that in none of the cases mentioned did it take more than three sessions to relieve the vomiting. Likewise, the root of the patient's emotional

SUMMARY OF COURSE OF TWELVE PATIENTS
WITH HYPEREMESIS GRAVIDARUM TREATED BY HYPNOSIS

Patient	Age	Period of Gestation	Number of Days of Severe Vomiting Prior to Initiation of Hypnotherapy	Emotional Problem	Number of Sessions of Hypnosis for Immediate Relief of Vomiting	Result of Pregnancy
F.G.	31	8 weeks	8	Homesickness	1	Full-term living female
A.R.	22	10 weeks	2	Domination by in-laws	1	Full-term living male
L.C.	25	6 weeks	4	Finances	2	Spontaneous abortion at 12 weeks
C.M.	21	11 weeks	6	Inadequate housing	1	Full-term living female
R.W.	29	5 weeks	3	Loss of career	2	Full-term living female
H.G.	31	7 weeks	4	Impending divorce	3	Full-term living male

SUMMARY OF COURSE OF TWELVE PATIENTS
WITH HYPEREMESIS GRAVIDARUM TREATED BY HYPNOSIS

Patient	Age	Period of Gestation	Number of Days of Severe Vomiting Prior to Initiation of Hypnotherapy	Emotional Problem	Number of Sessions of Hypnosis for Immediate Relief of Vomiting	Result of Pregnancy
A.S.	20	6 weeks	1	Inability to adjust to pregnancy	1	Full-term living female
M.B.	19	6 weeks	4	Aversion to pregnancy	1	Full-term living male
F.K.	25	8 weeks	6	Inadequate housing	1	Full-term living female
R.Q.	32	10 weeks	10	Did not want another child	1	Full-term living male
B.S.	34	12 weeks	4	Fear of pregnancy	1	Full-term living female
J.D.	24	10 weeks	3	Inadequate housing	1	Full-term living female

problem, in each instance, was speedily exposed with hypnosis.

Admittedly, the number of cases involved in this particular project was small. However, the doctors report, "it is encouraging to note that *all* patients benefited from this therapy. All the mothers recovered."

Our own research bears out the fact that, except in the most severe instances, patients suffering from nausea and vomiting always respond favorably to mild suggestive therapy and/or deeper hypnosis. In these cases, hypnosis hastens our insight into the causes of the difficulty, thereby speeding permanent relief. The patient, who at this point simply wants to feel well, is happy to accept this suggestion of well-being from a physician with whom a rapport has been established.

Heartburn

Approximately two thirds of all pregnant women suffer from heartburn. This may be described as a burning, or even scalding, sensation in the upper abdomen or lower part of the chest. Despite considerable research and investigation, the exact cause for this symptom is still not understood. We do know that the condition has nothing to do with the heart, despite our name for it. It appears to be, instead, a form of indigestion.

At one time, physicians believed that heartburn in pregnancy originated with the fetal mass pressing on the patient's stomach. This mistaken notion can still be heard around many bridge tables today. However, the truth of the matter is that, in the majority of cases, the symptom develops early in pregnancy when the uterus is still relatively small and incapable of causing any such discomfort. It is doubtful that even the fully-enlarged uterus, as indicated by the distorted stomach forced out of position, exerts the type of pressure that can cause this kind of distress.

What, then, is the origin of heartburn? And what can we do about it? To arrive at even a partial answer to these questions, we must turn to a study of heartburn by Drs. H. B. Tumen and E. M. Cohen in the *Journal of the American Medical Association* a decade ago. This study, involving both men and women, called attention to the personality make-up of those suffering from heartburn. Those individuals were found to be extremely tense, quick to anger, resentful, and easily offended. They were suspicious and prejudiced. This kept them on guard, so that relaxation was difficult. In addition, they were hard to get along with and critical of minor faults in others.

A recurring theme of this book is that our bodies are quite capable of expressing emotions, such as those just mentioned, in many physical ways. The selection of the esophagus and stomach as a showcase for such feelings in pregnancy cases may be regarded as evidence of the inability of the woman to "swallow" or "stomach" the pregnancy because of an unconscious aversion to it. For these reasons, the relief of anxiety and tensions is a very important part of the therapy for heartburn in pregnancy. With most women, the physician can accomplish this by the simplest of lessons in relaxation, coupled with a discussion and explanation of the harmlessness of the symptom, in order to allay the patient's fears. He may, also, through the use of posthypnotic suggestions, draw attention to the necessity for proper eating habits, ample time for meals, proper spacing of mealtimes, avoidance of eating while distracted, and avoidance of large meals and air-gulping.

Constipation

As a discomfort of pregnancy, constipation is especially important, because, if unchecked, it can develop into a more painful and troublesome case of hemorrhoids (clusters, at the opening of the rectum, of enlarged veins commonly called "piles"). In pregnancy, where the flow of blood to the area of the rectum is somewhat obstructed by the growing uterus, a patient is always susceptible to hemorrhoids unless the pressure in this region can be relieved by regular bowel movements.

There are many things you can do to assist regularity during pregnancy. A diet of leafy vegetables and fresh fruits will help, as will increased consumption of water. Your physician will have his own opinions regarding laxatives, and his advice should be heeded.

Our concern, for the moment, is with constipation as another item on the long list of psychosomatic manifestations of pregnancy. To understand some of the psychological causes for constipation, you may wish to recall our earlier discussion of the important "anal period" of infant development and the possible long-range effects of toilet training on the child. We have seen how either the passage or withholding of the feces creates pleasurable sensations during this time in our lives. To the child, who has not yet matured enough to look upon excreta as unclean or "disgusting," the attempts of her parents to regulate her bowel movements may be both confusing and frightening. Her very first lesson in this direction is all too frequently tied in with the fact that in order to obtain her mother's love and approval, she must restrict these movements. Sometimes this lesson is even more bitter, because the child quickly learns that she can express her own displeasure and hostility through the control (or lack of it) of excretory functions.

Thus, while passage of the feces may be pleasurable for the infant, withholding it for a less opportune time gives her a sense of power over her parents that she may not readily relinquish. Often, in the case of an adult woman, these conflicts will reappear in the form of constipation during pregnancy. These patients nearly always find it difficult to relax. They cling to the physician for protection, and they express an abnormal, almost childlike, concern for the type of anesthetic to be used during delivery.

Fortunately, the tensions usually respond very well to the relaxing therapy of hypnosis. The rapport thus established between doctor and patient, furthermore, lessens the patient's apprehensions of the delivery procedure. And, once again, we eliminate an undesirable behavior pattern.

Insomnia

Hypnosis is not sleep. As we have attempted to point out, it is, on the contrary, an even more alert state of awareness than the subject normally has. Yet hypnosis can materially assist you, especially during the latter part of your pregnancy, if you find it difficult to fall asleep. Naturally, there is an air of excitement over the forthcoming "event" that, in itself, will tend to keep you awake. And the movements of your baby within the uterus may be disturbing. Any one of a number of factors may contribute to your sleeplessness, but almost all of these can be dissolved with only a little effort and a firm, positive suggestion of sleep.

Insomnia, in normal cases of pregnancy, can be relieved by posthypnotic suggestion, autohypnosis, or a combination of the two. Sleep, after all, is largely a matter of habit. "I'm sleepy: it must be eleven o'clock" is a common way of telling time in many households. Our inability to fall asleep readily in strange surroundings is another sign of how habit-forming sleep can be.

By means of posthypnotic suggestion, we can refocus the subject's awareness on sleep-inducing habits to the exclusion of any disturbances other than those which pose a real physical threat. We often suggest to a hypnotized patient that, in the evening, at her regular hour for retiring or when she goes to bed, she will go into a natural, deep, relaxed sleep. This "sleep" is no different from any other. It does not alter the subject's capacity to awaken when she is fully rested or to respond to emergencies which may arise during the night.

With autohypnosis you can quickly fall asleep by giving yourself one of two totally different suggestions. In the first case, you merely relax yourself and suggest deep, refreshing sleep. This works well for a majority of subjects. In fact, most people use something like this to fall asleep at night without going through the formality of autohypnosis. Occasionally, however, it seems that the harder you try, even with hypnosis, the more difficult it is to fall asleep. Here, the second type of suggestion may be helpful. Instead of suggesting sleep, tell yourself that you will keep awake. It may be easier to do this if you pretend that you are a sentry manning a post at night or some other nighttime worker. No matter how you do it, try very hard to stay awake. Suggest to yourself: "My lids will remain open." Then, when your lids begin to blink, tell yourself that each time they blink, they will get heavier and heavier. Soon it will be difficult to stop them from blinking. By that time, you will be very happy to keep your eyes closed and let sleep come over you.

Overeating

The most obvious part of your pregnancy, of course, is the weight that you will be gaining. It would be impossible for you to have a normal, healthy baby without carrying around these additional pounds for six months or so. However, contrary to common gossip, there is no significant relationship between the weight you gain and the size of your baby. Nor does a large baby necessarily mean that you will have difficulty in delivery. All of this, however, should not imply permission to eat whatever and whenever you choose during pregnancy. If you overeat during pregnancy, you may still be paying the penalty for overweight long after your baby is born. At the very least, overeating causes more discomfort during pregnancy and greatly increases the possibility of complications prior to delivery.

You can expect to gain about twenty pounds before your baby arrives. This is a perfectly healthy sign. It represents the total weight of the baby, the afterbirth, the fluid surrounding the baby, the increases in the size of the uterus and breasts, and the accumulation of fluids in the body tissues.

Certainly you will not be gaining all of this at once. During the first three months of your pregnancy, your weight will remain fairly constant. Afterwards, you should gain an average of one pound a week until you reach the maximum weight for you, as determined by your physician. He will want to keep careful track of those extra pounds and will suggest certain changes in your diet to keep this increase in line. It will pay for you to follow his advice rather than some "rule of thumb," because no one can definitely say in advance how much weight you should gain. Then, too, there is a natural tendency in pregnancy to equalize overweight and underweight. That is, normally heavier women will tend to gain and retain proportionately less weight in childbearing than will slim women. In any case, provided that your increased weight is kept below the limit your doctor sets, the excess poundage will vanish within a week or two after delivery.

Remember that your doctor can do only so much. It is up to you to realize that you will not be quite so physically active as you were before becoming pregnant. Your daily requirements of energy-building foods will not be nearly as great. Those calories which you formerly burned almost as fast as you ate will now be stored as deposits of fat, unless there is a change in your eating habits. As we shall see, however, with the assistance of hypnosis this self-discipline need not be a difficult chore.

Some patients are faced with a much more serious problem. Instead of restricting their diets or even continuing to eat normally, they try to relieve anxiety-provoking tensions of childbirth by overeating. It is not too surprising that quite a few expectant mothers react in this manner. The seeds of habit are sown long before they become pregnant. Many women, usually capable of restraining their intake of food, are unable to do so during the premenstrual phase. Perhaps you were one of those who experienced increased irritation, tension, depression, or excitation at this time of the month. If so, you know that it is common for these emotional outbursts to bring with them an insatiable appetite for food before they disappear with the onset of menses.

No one knows exactly why this relationship between the tendency to overeat and the preceding irritations exists. But we have learned that glandular obesity is rare and that overweight is due to one simple fact—more food calories are being incorporated into the body than are being consumed by it.

"Of course I'm eating more, doctor," some women say. "After all, I'm eating for two." This very lame excuse for overindulgence in food is commonly heard from pregnant women who thrive on the sympathy of their husbands and families. Actually, it has little basis in fact. In order to maintain your health as well as that of your unborn child, you will need to eat and drink plenty of milk, cheese, eggs, and other protein-enriched foods. You will require, too, a substantial amount of sugar and starches. But the diet prescribed by your physician will be perfectly balanced in these vital ingredients with a minimum of calories.

The woman who falls back upon the "eating-for-two" excuse is generally failing to meet an adult situation on a mature level. Very likely, because she is not getting enough attention from those around her, she takes emotional refuge in the mother-love symbol of food. Subconsciously, she recalls how her parent expressed affection by setting a full plate before her. And how did she encourage and reciprocate this "love"? Why, by finishing every bit of that food, of course. This regression accounts, in part, for the fondness of the compulsive eater for sweets—a familiar bribe for "good" children in many households.

Occasionally we encounter an obstetric patient who, sensing the fact that she is tiring sooner than before, overeats because she feels that this will make up for the energy that she lacks. This self-therapy can be extremely dangerous, for the fatigue may indicate problems of an entirely different nature. For instance, it could result from simple anemia, low blood pressure, or some other difficulty that can best be managed by a physician. Even if we set such purely physical reasons aside for the moment, this "eating to keep up your strength" routine can be carried too far. One obese young patient, for example, admitted that she not only had three large meals a day but that she also loved to have an ice cream soda in the morning and a malted milk in the afternoon. In addition, she almost always had a bedtime snack and, between mealtimes, fortified herself with chocolate bars.

When this patient was asked why she behaved as she did, she replied: "Well, doctor, I really don't want to eat so much, but I get so darned hungry. If I missed a meal, I'd get so weak that I'd just collapse."

It was subsequently established through hypnoanalysis that the woman's eating habits were really convenient outlets for her emotions. When she was anxious, frightened, sad, or even happy, she would express herself through eating. With hypnotically-induced regression, she recalled that as a little girl she had been taught that food was a source of strength. She had to eat in order to "grow up to be a big, strong girl." Now, as an adult, the woman recognized that in order to conquer her obesity, she had to be strong. But this meant that in order to lose weight, she had to eat more. When the absurdity of the situation was explained to her, the patient gradually changed her attitude towards food until she was not only eating less but also enjoying what she ate more. For the first time in this woman's life, she recognized that food was something that could be tasted as well as chewed and that eating was more than mere stomach-stuffing.

Naturally, the average woman who neglects her weight does not go to the extremes just mentioned. If this is so, then, you might ask, "Why all this concern with over-eating?" The fact is that obesity is so common a problem in this country that it seems to be almost a way of life. It has been reliably estimated that there are more than twenty-five million overweight persons in the United States. Americans of both sexes are spending something around $250,000,000 annually on reducing pills, appliances, and reducing salons, most of which make hardly a dent in the waistline. The practices of some good physicians are con-fined almost exclusively to combating overweight with purely medicinal measures. Yet approximately forty per cent of these patients "fall off" their diets before treatment is con-cluded. Worse yet, a number of these obesity cases end up in the hands of nonmedical therapists, where they get lots of sympathy but little real assistance.

Aside from the money wasted, the price we pay for overeating is enormous. A recent study of fifty thousand overweight life-insurance policyholders revealed that those who were fifteen to twenty-four per cent heavier than aver-age for their builds had a forty-four per cent higher death rate resulting from a variety of direct causes. Additionally, impairment of the heart and kidney functions is more ap-parent in the overweight individual. Studies of a group of diabetics in a Boston, Massachusetts, hospital showed that eighty-five per cent of the patients were overweight, com-pared with just five per cent who were underweight.

We might go on to list a score of other chronic diseases which could result from your letting your weight "go" during pregnancy. However, we are primarily concerned here with overeating in the light of the harmful effects that this habit can have on your pregnancy and labor. These are no less considerable than are the long-range effects of carrying around too much weight. Obesity has definitely been linked with an increase in blood pressure, liver and kidney damage, and many of the poisonous complications of childbirth. Too often, abortion is nature's first line of defense against the development of such serious conditions. But even when the overweight woman is fortunate enough to escape this consequence, she may still needlessly suffer backaches and pains in the legs during the prenatal period. Such discomforts result from the strain of unnecessary weight on particular muscles.

Obviously, the immediate cause for overweight in pregnancy is overeating. No amount of drugs or psychology can change that fact. Furthermore, there is no known way to lose weight other than rigid dieting. This statement holds true even in the case of drug treatments for obesity, which have been moderately successful in recent years. Far from magically dissolving fat from the body, these drugs (basically amphetamines) inhibit the chemical secretions of the stomach, so that that organ remains full for a longer period. Another result of drug treatment is the sensation of well-being that the patient has, as opposed to the feeling of fatigue that, we have seen, commonly leads to overeating. No matter which result predominates, drug therapy, theoretically, leaves the patient feeling satisfied with her diet.

Your problem, therefore, if you tend to eat more than you should, is to find a good diet *and to stick to it*. We are not going to pretend that this is the easiest thing in the world to do. Many persons simply do not start dieting because they are afraid of failure.

In discussing the "obese personality," Dr. Hilde Bruch of

187

the Department of Psychiatry and Pediatrics, College of Physicians and Surgeons, Columbia University in New York City, observes that this type of individual is prone to set impossibly high goals for himself. "The person's inability to live up to his ambition is so great that he has to resort to some means of alleviating the tension and despair," Dr. Bruch says. "In fat people, overeating is the most important means of relieving the felt dissatisfaction. It fulfills the primitive hope that eating will make up for the defect. Yet, however much food they take, eating never gives the satisfaction they really want to feel. It does not accomplish the very special things they want to accomplish. The resulting increase in size fulfills, on a primitive symbolic level, the desire to be big."

As if this were not enough, society seems to go out of its way to make life very difficult for the person who sincerely wants to lose weight. Food and drink, as signs of affection or as incentives to love, are symbolic of most social entertaining. Even if she wants to resist temptation, the overweight individual may fear that refusal of these offerings will be interpreted as rejection of the host's "love." In the business world, food has assumed a role far out of proportion to its nutritional value. The best business "deals" are often made over a well-laid table, and it is considered poor taste for either the host or his guest to permit the other to eat or drink alone. Finally, diets can be very disturbing to the family routine, particularly when they involve special food preparations for one member of the group. The interpersonal struggles over eating habits that absorb some families make many youngsters everlastingly resistant to the very word "dieting."

Unfortunately, there is no pat solution to these problems. Besides recommending a good diet, your physician can guide you around some of the pitfalls along the pathway of dieting. He might even point out the difference between the pangs of the genuine hunger for food and those of the psychological hunger that comes from such things as the memory of the "fun" of eating. Still, it is up to you, the patient, to take the final, determined step.

You can best accomplish this, not by an exercise of will power to refrain from overeating, but by experiencing an overwhelming desire to be thin. This fixity of purpose—a concentration of awareness upon reducing—should remind you of our earlier definition of hypnosis. The principle is the same, no matter what you call the procedure.

Reducing is one of the most effective uses of autohypnosis. This is precisely what movie actor Cary Grant meant when he told an interviewer that he manages to keep his slim figure by "thinking thin." Countless less-celebrated subjects are employing the same technique with equally good results. Specifically, if the subject, with autohypnosis or the assistance of her hypnotist, can regress to a period when she was not so fat and keep this self-image uppermost in her mind, she will *want* to lose weight. To fortify this picture, the subject may find it helpful to use some rather unusual devices. One patient, for example, bought a beautiful dress a size too small and hung it on the door of the bathroom, where she could see it at the start of each day of dieting.

If you really want to keep yourself slender, you will find hypnosis a useful tool in a number of ways. Aside from suggesting autohypnosis, we frequently use the phenomenon of posthypnotic suggestion to inculcate better eating habits. After achieving a medium to deep state of relaxation, the subject is requested to think of the most disgusting, loathsome, and revolting smell or taste she can imagine. Everyone has at least one food which he naturally dislikes and the thought of which readily stimulates such images. The suggestion is made that every time the subject eats forbidden food or even thinks about breaking her diet, she will develop the same nauseating smell and taste associated with the disliked food.

Secondly, it is suggested that, henceforth, each and every bit of liquid or solid food consumed will be rolled from the tip of the tongue to the back of the mouth and from side to side. The purpose of this suggestion is to give all of the taste cells or buds on the tongue a chance to savor the food. Since besides eating ravenously, most obese persons bolt their food, it may be expected that if they eat slowly and get maximum enjoyment out of each mouthful, they will realize greater satisfaction from less food intake.

As effective as autohypnosis or posthypnotic suggestions may be for a time, hypnosis alone cannot permanently cure the overeating habit. The subject's understanding of her emotional impulses and their relationship to her attitude towards food is. an essential ingredient for all successful dieting. Some patients manage to achieve this insight simply by inquiring into their own motives for overeating; most require some sort of help. With this larger, latter group, hypnoanalysis has been particularly helpful in getting the patient to *want truly* to reduce.

Cravings

Contemporary literature is so full of the "pickles and ice cream" symptom of pregnancy that it is no wonder that our young women grow up expecting to have cravings for unusual foodstuffs while they are bearing children. If you are pregnant, you do not have to "crave" anything. Indeed, the number of patients who do actually suffer this particular discomfort is very small when compared with, say, the number who overeat. On the other hand, those who experience cravings may demand anything from out-of-season fruits to other difficult-to-get or bizarre combinations of foods. Instances have been reported where pregnant women craved chalk, slate pencils, clay, salt, or sand. There is even a case on record where an otherwise perfectly normal patient craved a bite of her husband's arm—and took it.

Happily, the more unusual cravings are extremely rare. The majority of women who make strange demands at all are apparently content with requesting foods which keep their husbands scurrying about in neighborhood stores at all hours of the day and night. And this need for attention is probably the real reason that cravings exist—because they cannot be explained by any physical changes occurring in the expectant mother during pregnancy. Instead, the symptom nearly always indicates a faulty psychosexual development leading to childish notions of making the husband suffer for his role in conceiving the baby. These immature emotions, too, reflect an almost childlike fear of going through with childbirth.

Against this emotional background, whenever "cravings" reach the discomfort stage or the point where the patient herself wants to do something about them, hypnoanalysis and hypnotherapy can be most effective in providing relief. For example, while she represents a very small minority of all pregnant women, the expectant mother who is emotionally ill-prepared for her forthcoming role and who subconsciously wishes to punish herself for becoming pregnant is not a stranger to us. This woman may try to alleviate her feelings of guilt by eating large amounts of food or even objects that she considers harmful. However, when, with hypnosis, her awareness is concentrated upon more healthy aspects of her pregnancy, the cravings almost always cease.

Miscarriage

Abortion, or "miscarriage," as the condition is commonly called, remains one of the most serious problems of pregnancy that some patients and obstetricians must face. Despite our very considerable gains in conditioning women to normal, healthy childbearing, an estimated two hundred thousand babies in this country each year are born too early for survival. These are spontaneous abortions, with the birth occurring prior to the seventh month of pregnancy, before the baby is sufficiently developed to live outside of the mother's body. Actually, our figures tell us only part of the unfortunate story, because they do not include an undetermined number of both "therapeutic" abortions induced by reputable physicians to protect the life of the mother and "criminal" abortions performed by a very small group of people all too eager to prey on the miseries of some women.

At the moment, honest medical research is much concerned with the questions of why spontaneous abortions happen and how they may be prevented. Some doctors, seizing upon the fact that well over fifty per cent of the aborted embryos are defective in one way or another, hold that the abortion is simply nature's way of getting rid of an imperfect creation. Others report a degree of success in preventing miscarriages through the administration of Vitamins C and K, thyroid extracts, sedatives, and other drugs. Still other physicians prescribe complete bed rest and abstinence from sexual intercourse at the very first sign of difficulty. Almost all, though, agree that freedom from anxiety over the pregnancy is important in preventing miscarriages.

One of the most outstanding features of these spontaneous abortions is that they tend to occur more frequently in cases where the patient has a history of interrupted pregnancies. In fact, it may be said that some women develop an "abortion habit," just as some of us seem to be "addicted to" accidents. An analysis, not too long ago, of six thousand miscarriages indicated that if a woman has had a previous abortion, her chances of not repeating it are seventy-eight per cent. With two previous consecutive abortions, her chances drop to sixty-two per cent. With three, they are twenty-seven per cent. With four, the likelihood of the patient's not repeating is only six per cent. In many of the cases studied, the development of the embryo up to the time of miscarriage was perfectly normal.

We cannot be certain at this time why some women, despite the best medical care and attention, are habitual aborters and why others seem to go blithely on their pregnant ways ignoring even severe physical shocks. There is, however, strong reason to suspect that maternal emotional instability plays an important role in miscarriages. You can follow this line of reasoning quite easily if you consider what emotional trials do to the childbearing habits of animals. Chickens, for instance, drop their eggs and molt when frightened. Certain domestic animals, when exposed to the vicissitudes of wildlife, experience difficulty in carrying their young. But when these same animals are protected, with many of these dangers eliminated, they carry to term and their litters increase.

In humans the effects of unpleasant experiences on the tenacity of certain muscles are even more apparent, because these effects are often accompanied by such revealing remarks as "it makes my hair stand on end" and "it grips me." When these disturbances, which originate with fear and anxiety, react upon the sympathetic nerves to the bladder and intestines, we hear: "I was so frightened, I almost wet my pants." It is not unreasonable, therefore, to suspect that other organs of the body (specifically the uterus) can become involved in the chain of reactions caused by an emotional problem.

It is highly unlikely that your pregnancy will end in a miscarriage. Even if you are one of those abortion-prone individuals we mentioned earlier, it is probable that merely the strong and positive assurance from your physician that your pregnancy *will be* maintained can break this distressing habit. No matter how you accomplish it, your first goal should be to eliminate the doubts and fears you might have concerning your ability to have a healthy delivery. If you can attain this objective, there will be far less chance of these fears' being transmitted to the muscles around your uterus, which can contract enough to loosen or disturb the placental circulation so necessary for nourishment of the growing embryo.

Hypnosis can help! By assisting the patient to concentrate upon the healthy activities of her mind and muscles, it brings to bear all of her resources for a successful pregnancy. Even without direct suggestion, the tenseness of the subject vanishes—as is evidenced by real physical changes, such as reduction in blood pressure and variations in metabolic activity. We have had occasion to use hypnotherapy with several pregnant women who developed signs and symptoms of abortion. After these women were put in a state of "deep sleep" for twelve to fifteen hours and then awakened naturally, they reported no signs of the tensions, anxieties, and abdominal cramps that had bothered them earlier. All were trained in autohypnosis and carried through to a normal, healthy delivery.

CHAPTER X

•

Your Doctor and Hypnosis

"Nothing should be omitted in an art which interests the whole world, one which may be beneficial to suffering humanity and which does not risk human life or comfort."

Hippocrates

BOON TO MANKIND . . . or witchcraft!

Today, a full century after Dr. Esdaile used hypnoanesthesia to perform hundreds of successful operations upon illiterate natives of India and over two thousand years after the physicians of Eastern Europe and the Near East first employed suggestion to alleviate suffering, there are still many competent medical men who honestly cannot make up their minds about using hypnosis in their practices. And because physicians are, after all, only human, there is even a small group who would condemn the use of hypnosis without giving the technique a fair trial. Fortunately, as the subject is incorporated into more medical texts, mentioned repeatedly in professional journals, and discussed more and more at medical association gatherings, the number of dissenters is decreasing rapidly.

However, to you, as a patient, the attitude of *your* doctor towards the subject should be of paramount importance in deciding whether or not you will permit hypnosis to benefit you. This is true of any medical procedure. But it is especially so in the case of hypnosis because, as we have stated, the success of the technique hinges upon the establishment of a rapport between the doctor/hypnotist and the patient/subject. In other words, the two must, literally and figuratively, "speak the same language."

We cannot say for certain what position your physician takes on the subject of hypnosis. But we do know what reputable members of the profession are saying about the value of suggestion, generally, and hypnosis, specifically. These opinions are those of scientifically-oriented men who are neither particularly anxious to associate themselves with a fad nor so bound by tradition that they cannot accept progress in any direction. Furthermore, their attitudes are based upon considerable research. The report of the Council on Mental Health (a committee of the American Medical Association), for example, represents a two-year study of the use of hypnosis in medicine and is the result of interviews with doctors and dentists who have spent a good part of their careers studying the relationship of hypnosis to the welfare and comfort of their patients. A study of some of these comments should assist you in establishing a common meeting ground with your own physician.

MEDICAL USE OF HYPNOSIS

Excerpts from a report approved by the Board of Trustees and the House of Delegates of the American Medical Association at its June 1958 meeting in San Francisco, California.

"The history of hypnosis since the time of Mesmer has been characterized by a series of curious cycles alternating between great interest and almost complete rejection. This phenomenon in itself is an indication of the somewhat mystical aura that has surrounded the subject throughout the years. Recently, owing to a concatenation of circumstances, there has been a reawakened interest in hypnosis. In part, the experiences of World War II contributed to this interest.

"The Council on Mental Health of the American Medical Association has for some years received numerous inquiries from physicians throughout the United States relating to the subject of hypnosis, many of them asking for information regarding training programs in this area. A group of serious workers in medicine has been reporting on various aspects of the utilization of hypnosis. In addition, the dental profession has become interested in its use in relation to its own practice. Concurrently, "fringe" groups have been exploiting hypnosis through the press, radio, and television. Overpopularization in this as in other areas of medicine usually leads to oversimplification. Overdramatized events are seized on to the general detriment of sober scientific work.

". . . The work of the Hypnosis Committee was limited to the specific theme of the medical use of hypnosis in its therapeutic aspects, since this seemed to be the most relevant area for the Council's consideration. . . . The Committee emphasized certain regressive aspects of hypnosis. It also stressed the fact that hypnotic phenomena were of a wide variety and should not be limited only to the so-called trance state.

"In order to begin to understand these phenomena it is necessary to place hypnosis within the general framework of psychodynamic psychology and psychiatry. . . . In a sense it is unfortunate that the induction of hypnosis is generally so simple a matter that it requires little or no technical skill or training. This, in itself, represents one of the main hazards in its utilization, since it lends itself to oversimplification and overdramatization with a production of spectacular phenomena that are meat for the charlatan.

". . . Hypnosis should be used on a highly selective basis by such individuals [persons who are qualified by background and training] and should never become a single technique used under all circumstances by a therapist. No physician or dentist should utilize hypnosis for purposes that are not related to his particular specialty and that are beyond the range of his ordinary competence. As an example, a trained and qualified dentist might use hypnosis for hypnoanesthesia or hypnoanalgesia or for the allaying of anxiety in relation to specific dental work. Under no circumstances would it be proper for him to use hypnosis for the treatment of neurotic difficulties of his patient. The surgeon, obstetrician, anesthesiologist, gynecologist, internist, and general practitioner may legitimately utilize these techniques within the framework of their own particular field of competence.

". . . Certain aspects of hypnosis still remain unknown and controversial, as is true in many other areas of medicine and the psychological sciences. Therefore, active participation in high-level research by members of the medical and dental professions is to be encouraged. The use of hypnosis for entertainment purposes is vigorously condemned."

MEDICAL USE OF HYPNOTISM
(British Report)

Excerpts from a report of a subcommittee appointed in November 1953 by the Psychological Medicine Group Committee of the British Medical Association.

". . . The hypnotic state may be described as follows: "A temporary condition of altered attention in the subject which may be induced by another person and in which a variety of phenomena may appear spontaneously or in response to verbal or other stimuli. These phenomena include alterations in consciousness and memory, increased susceptibility to suggestion, and the production in the subject of responses and ideas unfamiliar to him in his usual state of mind. Further, phenomena such as anesthesia, paralysis and rigidity of muscles, and vasomotor changes can be produced and removed in the hypnotic state.

"There is a wide range of hypnotic manifestations which are by no means confined to the so-called trance. If all types of phenomena are taken into account it may be stated that the majority of people can be hypnotized, but in only a minority is it possible to induce a deep trance in a single session.

"Like other remedies hypnotism has its indications and contraindications, and considerable knowledge and expert judgement are required to decide when hypnotism is likely to help the patient, and whether it should be used by itself or as a complement to other methods of psychotherapy. For these reasons the Subcommittee is of the opinion that hypnotism should not be regarded as a specialty independent of psychological medicine.

". . . The dangers of hypnotism have been exaggerated in some quarters. The Subcommittee is convinced, however, that they do exist, especially when it is used without proper consideration of persons predisposed, constitutionally or by the effects of disease, to severe psychoneurotic reactions or antisocial behaviour.

". . . Hypnotism may involve the rapid or immediate development of a relationship between hypnotist and subject of the same order and intensity as is produced more slowly in the course of psychotherapy. . . . It is recommended, therefore, that the use of hypnotism in the treatment of physical and psychological disorders should be confined to persons subscribing to the recognized ethical code which governs the relation of doctor and patient. This would not preclude its use by a suitably trained psychologist or medical auxiliary of whose competence the medical practitioner was personally satisfied, and who would carry out, under medical direction, the treatment of patients selected by the physician.

"Instruction in the clinical use of hypnotism should be

given to all medical postgraduates training as specialists in psychological medicine, and possibly, say, to trainee anesthetists and obstetricians, so that they will understand its indications and practical applications. The Subcommittee holds that no special 'gift' is required to induce it: there are various techniques of equal efficacy.

". . . Since hypnotism very readily produces an intense relationship between patient and doctor it provides a means of research into the general problem of the patient-doctor relationship. Further, because of the relative brevity of treatment with hypnotism, such research may contribute to a solution of the problem created by the very large number of people requiring psychotherapy, and this possibility should be explored in the clinical field."

PAINLESS LABOR

Excerpts of opinions of the late Dr. Joseph B. DeLee, Professor of Obstetrics, University of Chicago Medical School, and Chief of Obstetrics, Chicago Lying-In Hospital.

"May it be that we are depriving women of an emotional experience which they need to complete their life, indeed to prevent certain psychologic reactions, similar to the results of frustration of desire?

"In this respect a painless labor would be similar to an interrupted orgasm, and we do not need to have the psychoanalysts tell us what follows these disturbed functions. If you were to lay this matter before the women, most of them would pooh-pooh it, but they do lots of things that are not good for them, and scoff at our warnings. Actually, I have often felt that the women miss something when they are delivered under a chemical anesthetic—the thrill of hearing their baby's first cry. Labor must be tame for these women; but they seem to like it this way, and we of the medical profession must make it safe for them.

". . . All analgesics and general anesthetics are protoplasmic poisons of varying degree and affect the brain, nerve centers, heart, liver, et al.; they all affect the baby likewise. Our object in using them is to prevent the pain sensations arising in the pelvis from reaching the sensorium [the sensory apparatus of the brain]. Now pain can reach the sensorium in another way; through the mind. With our drugs, we try to prevent this too; but as was said, all drugs have inherent dangers.

". . . Therefore, we must block the only other route to the sensorium. There are two ways: drugs again, and suggestion, even a mild hypnotism or a combination of both. If we invoke the woman's mind, we can reduce the amount of drugging or dispense with it entirely. This depends mainly on the physician—to a much less extent on the patient. If you have what Solomon called 'an understanding heart,' you will be successful with local anesthesia."

HYPNOSIS

Pertinent quotes from an editorial which appeared in the September-October 1957 issue of the Western Journal of Surgery, Obstetrics and Gynecology.

". . . Our modern day technics of hypnosis—mesmerism's current form—have been so improved and simplified that this clinical method has become a very challenging and useful tool again within recent years. Unfortunately, it is a method which has been subject to a great deal of sensationalism, misinterpretation and false claims.

"A mother singing a lullaby to her child is a frequent and familiar example of hypnosis of a very practical nature. Mary Baker Eddy, the founder of the Christian Science religion, was a hypnotist of ability before she cloaked her technics with the legitimacy of Theology. Many physicians use this agent—Christian Science—in the care of the terminal cancer patient with intractable pain. Self-hypnosis of this kind under these circumstances may be most sparing. When the physician walks into the sickroom, his very presence and air of authority give very real assistance to the sick person.

". . . Esdaile stated in 1846, 'Mesmerism often comes to the aid of my patients when all the resources of medicine are exhausted and all the drugs of Arabia useless; and therefore, I consider it to be my duty to benefit by it.'

"Hypnosis has come a far cry from those days. It now is applicable not simply to pain relief itself but to a general inquiry into the basic physiological and psychological problems of our patients' bodies. It would seem most worthwhile for any conscientious practitioner to be as curious as Esdaile in the behalf of his patient."

Robert N. Rutherford, M.D.
Seattle, Washington

RELAXATION THROUGH HYPNOSIS

Portions of an address presented to the American Dental Society of Anesthesiology, Miami Beach, Florida, November 3, 1957.

"On numerous occasions I have talked with both physicians and dentists who have taken courses of instruction in hypnosis but who are afraid to use it because of the possible criticism of their own patients and other members of their professions.

"Many of these men believe that they would have the courage to use hypnosis if they could change its name, and some do so. It is my opinion that if hypnosis is intelligently explained to an intelligent patient, names are of no great importance. I tell my patients that hypnosis as used in medicine and dentistry is quite·different from that used by the stage hypnotist in concept, method of induction, and, of course, in application.

". . . One of the first things I tell the patient is that hypnosis is a restful, enjoyable, relaxed state, and that I am going to teach him how to relax. I impress upon him that hypnosis is entirely a cooperative effort, that the doctor is the teacher and leader, but that for the most part, he, the subject, really hypnotizes himself. He must understand that the extent to which he enters the hypnotic state is largely dependent on his own ability to relax, and his acceptance of and response to suggestions.

"I inform the patient that I will use the word 'sleep,' and that he will close his eyes, but that he will not really be asleep. He will be conscious, and aware of his surroundings, and what is being said to him. The word 'sleep' is used merely to give him an idea of the relaxed state he will enter.

". . . Relaxation through hypnosis is a learning process. The subject becomes a better subject as he learns what is expected of him. This is the reason a person becomes an increasingly better subject the second, third or tenth time he undergoes hypnosis—not that his mind has been weakened or controlled.

". . . While in trance the patient closes his eyes and goes deeper into trance. He takes a deep breath, and as he exhales the air from his lungs, he goes deeper and continues to go deeper as various parts of his body become more and more relaxed, and he accepts more and more of the doctor's suggestions."

Lawrence Milton Staples, D.M.D.
Visiting Instructor
Tufts University School of
Dental Medicine

There are any number of precedents from all branches of medicine for your physician to follow if he is truly objective about the use of hypnosis. Of all the uses to which the procedure has been put, the relief of discomfort and pain in childbirth is, perhaps, the easiest for the individual trained in other facets of medicine to master. In this regard, hypnosis is only a valuable tool—it might be compared to a scalpel. Every physician can be taught how to hold a scalpel to make an incision into the abdomen, but once the operation has begun it takes a man with years of training to know what to do with that scalpel. Likewise, hypnosis, when used for purposes other than inducing relaxation and anesthesia—for example, psychotherapy—requires a broad knowledge of psychologic techniques.

Our attention in this chapter is directed towards your obstetrician, who can deliver perfectly beautiful babies safely without qualifying as a psychoanalyst. Of course, he will want to know as much about your personality as he can—why you wish to have painless labor, how much you are going to depend upon him, and how much relief you expect from pain-relieving agents. Last, but far from least, he will try to determine how badly you really wish to have a baby and whether or not you are desirous of participating in the moment of its birth.

In so far as anesthesia is concerned, neither you nor your

physician need have any fear that any responsible individual is trying to "sell" hypnosis as a substitute for present-day methods of anesthesia, although hypnosis does have definite preoperative and postoperative advantages. Every doctor knows that reassurance and support, the mainstays of therapy for alleviating any acute psychological crisis, are also important in preparing a patient for anesthesia. We are merely contending, in addition, that such support can be rendered more rapidly by suggestive relaxation. With balanced anesthesia—that is, chemoanesthesia combined with hypnosis—it is possible to lessen the quantity of drugs used in labor and delivery by fifty to seventy-five per cent. A very real result of this "balanced approach" is the reduction of fetal anoxia among newborn infants by as much as eighty-five per cent, especially when inhalation anesthesia is eliminated.

Another reason we advocate the use of hypnosis by your physician is that this simple procedure can be a valuable adjunct in alleviating the fear, tension, and apprehension associated with childbirth and other more complicated surgical procedures. In the case of the Caesarean hysterectomy mentioned in an earlier chapter, the patient saw her nine-and-three-quarter-pound infant delivered and considered the whole experience a most satisfying one. At no time was she in pain, and, in spite of considerable surgery and loss of blood, no sign of shock was evident.

We have delivered several hundred mothers by either pure hypnosis or a combination of hypnosis and chemoanesthesia. About twenty to twenty-five per cent of these patients, carefully chosen for their high degree of susceptibility to suggestion, were carried through the first and second stages of labor without analgesia or anesthesia. Fifty per cent of all of our patients required only minimal amounts of sedation, usually near the end of the first stage. Local anesthesia was used for the episiotomy and repair. Even if you consider the remaining twenty-five per cent— and remember that this smaller group includes abnormal labors—failures, hypnotically speaking, of course, the results are still worth the effort. *All* of our patients benefit, to a degree, by learning about hypnosis, because they are better equipped to face the emotional trials of motherhood.

Hypnosis is used only at the patient's request. And we are careful not to make a woman feel guilty if she has to ask for anesthesia. But we are constantly trying to improve our techniques to increase the number of women who can benefit from hypnosis. Our results have been better, for example, since we instituted group hypnotic training. There seems to be an "emotional contagion" in a group, primarily because no woman likes to feel that another woman is better than she. Also, there is a group identification factor, wherein all members are trying to please the obstetrician.

Your physician should be aware that there is not the remotest possibility of danger from actual hypnotic induction, except, as we have stated elsewhere, if it is applied to severely disturbed patients. But this is a risk which the medical practitioner takes every day of his career. It is inherently present in every doctor/patient relationship whether or not hypnosis is used.

Every obstetrician has to be confident of his authority and prestige. Basic elements are necessary to establish rapport with his patient quickly. As a matter of fact, your doctor is constantly using suggestion, verbally or nonverbally, as part of his "bedside manner." Hypnosis is simply the scientific application of these same basic suggestions. It is well known among physicians, nurses, and other attendants of the woman in labor that the very presence of the obstetrician in the labor and delivery room is the equivalent of a half grain of morphine and is certainly conducive to producing relaxation in the patient, who has supreme confidence in "her" doctor. In this respect, too, every practicing obstetrician is consciously or unconsciously utilizing some form of suggestion at all times.

APPENDIX

"Dear doctor,

"As you so often stated, the entire experience was so very exciting, and being able to take an active part in the delivery of my child through hypnosis was truly an exciting and gratifying emotional experience for me.

"It is extremely difficult to describe the exhilaration which I felt at the climax of the delivery. It was a feeling which I wish strongly that every mother could experience. Truly, it was one of the most memorable events in my life. If the opportunity presents itself again, I will be most eager to use my past experience as a guide, and would once more make use of hypnosis in childbirth." ——Mrs. C.N.

•

"My water broke about 1:30 A.M. At first, I got the shakes, but then calmed down by doing some dishes and relaxing. I went to the hospital, and by a quarter to three I was prepared, and in the delivery room. The girl in the next room was in labor too, and fighting it every inch of the way with loud protests. This unnerved me at first, but I tried not to think of it, and managed to relax. After fifteen or twenty minutes, I wanted to bear down. It seemed far too soon to start pushing, but there was no stopping it.

"Then, my doctor said, 'O.K., you're ready to deliver. Let's get nice and relaxed.' I cooperated immediately. By the count of ten, I was relaxed. As I was lowering my stiffened arm, I had about my fourth or fifth contraction where I felt like pushing violently, but there was no pain. I heard my doctor say, 'Open your eyes. One more push, and you will have the baby.' I thought he was kidding, but with the next contraction, the baby was born. I looked at her, and exclaimed, 'It's amazing. This is easier than having a tooth pulled.'

"As they were putting in my last stitches, just an hour and a half after arriving at the hospital, the nurse whispered to me to look at the sunrise. I turned my head to view the colors, and thought what a fitting end to the beautiful experience of having my firstborn with hypnosis." ——Mrs. J.M.

•

"In May, I had the most thrilling experience of my life. I gave birth to a baby daughter without any chemical anesthesia. I had thought that I wanted some, but when I was refused, because the doctor knew the baby would be born in a minute, I was so grateful that I was able to experience her birth fully conscious and aware of when her head and shoulders came.

"The method used for my labor contractions and delivery was a form of deep to medium relaxation and breathing exercises for which I had been in training for about seven months. I can say with full authority—'I know it helped.' I had two other babies by spinal anesthesia with no foreknowledge of breathing exercises, and without knowing a way to relax. As a result, during both those previous times, I was tense, fearful, uncooperative, and had prolonged labor with slow recoveries.

"What a difference! During this pregnancy, I had not one sick or uncomfortable moment. I looked forward with joy—not dread—to the birth. When the contractions started,

I was able to cooperate, and count the breaths as I was told to do. When, a short time later, during delivery, I was told to bear down, again I was able to cooperate. My doctor was with me at all times; talking soothingly, helping me to relax, and to go into a mild hypnotic state. This entire wonderful pregnancy and delivery I attribute directly to the classes in learning about hypnotism, and deep relaxation." ——Mrs. D.N.

•

"Having my baby with the help of hypnosis was a very thrilling experience for me. I was able to watch the delivery, and was free from anxiety and fear. Since this was to be my first child, I wanted, mainly, to be able to relax enough at the time of delivery so that I could work along with each contraction, as the doctor taught us, instead of tightening up with fear.

"My baby was delivered, without any drugs or anesthetic within two hours and forty minutes after I reached the hospital. I feel that the instructions I received at the doctor's classes both in hypnosis, and in what to expect during labor played an important part in making me comfortable."
——Mrs. P.B.

•

"On August —, I gave birth to a 6 pound 13½ ounce baby boy while under hypnosis, and it was a memorable experience. Having had practically no illness during my childhood, I had developed a fear of doctors and hospitals. Yet, due to the conditioning period during my maternity visits to the doctor's office, I entered the hospital with absolutely no nervous feeling of any kind in connection with the delivery.

"The personal attention of my doctor, such as his use of my first name, helped create the feeling of self-confidence, and assurance that I could overcome my phobias. Knowing that the doctor and my husband would be present during the labor period also gave me an added feeling of relaxation.

"The hypnosis, in my case, was administered via the telephone during the first stages of labor. Though I was not in a private labor room, and had to witness other women's reactions, I still did not feel any apprehension. I had a sense of detachment. Though the pain was present, my body was relaxed. I was fully aware of the surroundings, and was able to inquire, while in the delivery room, as to the sex of my baby, and whether he was in good health. A complete feeling of exhilaration followed the birth of my child, and, after a four-day stay at the hospital, I returned home feeling well and happy.

"Four years later, I gave birth to my second son, 6 pounds 11½ ounces. This delivery, with hypnosis, was even more effective, because of the confidence I had developed from my first child's birth. I saw my son immediately after he was born, in the delivery room. It was a thrill a mother never forgets. This time, I was out of bed almost immediately, and in three days I returned home." ——Mrs. M.E.

●

"I am one of those persons who go through mental torture at the thought of any kind of physical pain, so naturally the thought of having a baby really frightened me. I think every woman has, at some time, read in books, or heard from other women how the mother suffers in childbirth.

"My first visit with the doctor helped to eliminate a few fears, when he explained that the birth process is a normal function, and that, with the use of hypnosis, my fears could be eased. He told me how my child's birth could be made easier for both of us. During my other prenatal visits, he began conditioning me, through the use of hypnosis, to accept his suggestions that I could feel no pain, and that I could be completely relaxed.

"The birth of my son was an enriching experience. When I arrived at the hospital at 1:00 A.M., the labor contractions were just beginning. My doctor came at once. He simply talked to me quietly, constantly repeating the suggestion that I would feel no pain. I could feel the contractions shake my body, but they were not painful. I was aware of the progress of my labor, but was able to relax, and talk with my husband.

"When I was taken to the delivery room, I was conscious, but relaxed deeply enough to reduce the physical sensations, and able to help the birth. The baby arrived at 5:55 A.M. I had some anesthetic for the afterbirth, but when I was taken down to my room I felt alive and very elated. My child was born after a shorter period of labor than most first babies, and I feel that this was due to the use of hypnosis." —Mrs. A.R.

•

"Because my doctor could not be present at the time of my baby's delivery, I had to rely on self-hypnosis. Frankly, I was unsuccessful during my first stage of labor, because the hospital obstetrics ward was overcrowded, and I was unable to concentrate. When the pains became almost unbearable, I decided it was up to me entirely to relieve the pain with hypnosis. I went to the only place where I could be alone—the bathroom.

"In less than one minute of intense concentration, the

pain was completely gone, and my second stage of labor started almost immediately thereafter. From that time on, the only sensation I had was a tremendous pushing feeling, and an uncomfortable urge to grunt, and push as hard as possible. In the delivery room, I was able to watch my baby's birth through a large mirror. It was the most exciting and satisfying experience of my life. I would never consider having a baby any other way." ——Mrs. R.K.

•

"I find myself amused at the doubts and frustrations I experienced during attendance at your classes, and in my experiments with self-hypnosis at home. You see, I tried to make more of a mystery of hypnosis than it really is. I must even confess that I was disappointed when I first discovered that there was no 'magic' involved. The doubts arose when I found that I had to depend upon myself to bring about the state of hypnosis, and the frustration of having no 'gauge' to measure by.

"My doctor, though, provided me with a satisfactory explanation of what hypnosis really is, when, during the last few moments of labor, he mentioned how nice it is for a patient to have training in 'self-discipline.' That's truly what it is, and how enlightening it was for me to have found that 'key.'" ——Mrs. R.B.

•

A Personal Word From Melvin Powers
Publisher, Wilshire Book Company

Dear Friend:

My goal is to publish interesting, informative, and inspirational books. You can help me accomplish this by answering the following questions, either by phone or by mail. Or, if convenient for you, I would welcome the opportunity to visit with you in my office and hear your comments in person.

Did you enjoy reading this book? Why?

Would you enjoy reading another similar book?

What idea in the book impressed you the most?

If applicable to your situation, have you incorporated this idea in your daily life?

Is there a chapter that could serve as a theme for an entire book? Please explain.

If you have an idea for a book, I would welcome discussing it with you. If you already have one in progress, write or call me concerning possible publication. I can be reached at (213) 875-1711 or (213) 983-1105.

Sincerely yours,

Melvin Powers

12015 Sherman Road
North Hollywood, California 91605

MELVIN POWERS SELF-IMPROVEMENT LIBRARY

ASTROLOGY

____ASTROLOGY: HOW TO CHART YOUR HOROSCOPE *Max Heindel*	3.00
____ASTROLOGY: YOUR PERSONAL SUN-SIGN GUIDE *Beatrice Ryder*	3.00
____ASTROLOGY FOR EVERYDAY LIVING *Janet Harris*	2.00
____ASTROLOGY MADE EASY *Astarte*	3.00
____ASTROLOGY MADE PRACTICAL *Alexandra Kayhle*	3.00
____ASTROLOGY, ROMANCE, YOU AND THE STARS *Anthony Norvell*	4.00
____MY WORLD OF ASTROLOGY *Sydney Omarr*	5.00
____THOUGHT DIAL *Sydney Omarr*	4.00
____WHAT THE STARS REVEAL ABOUT THE MEN IN YOUR LIFE *Thelma White*	3.00

BRIDGE

____BRIDGE BIDDING MADE EASY *Edwin B. Kantar*	7.00
____BRIDGE CONVENTIONS *Edwin B. Kantar*	5.00
____BRIDGE HUMOR *Edwin B. Kantar*	5.00
____COMPETITIVE BIDDING IN MODERN BRIDGE *Edgar Kaplan*	4.00
____DEFENSIVE BRIDGE PLAY COMPLETE *Edwin B. Kantar*	10.00
____GAMESMAN BRIDGE—Play Better with Kantar *Edwin B. Kantar*	5.00
____HOW TO IMPROVE YOUR BRIDGE *Alfred Sheinwold*	3.00
____IMPROVING YOUR BIDDING SKILLS *Edwin B. Kantar*	4.00
____INTRODUCTION TO DEFENDER'S PLAY *Edwin B. Kantar*	3.00
____SHORT CUT TO WINNING BRIDGE *Alfred Sheinwold*	3.00
____TEST YOUR BRIDGE PLAY *Edwin B. Kantar*	5.00
____VOLUME 2—TEST YOUR BRIDGE PLAY *Edwin B. Kantar*	5.00
____WINNING DECLARER PLAY *Dorothy Hayden Truscott*	4.00

BUSINESS, STUDY & REFERENCE

____CONVERSATION MADE EASY *Elliot Russell*	3.00
____EXAM SECRET *Dennis B. Jackson*	3.00
____FIX-IT BOOK *Arthur Symons*	2.00
____HOW TO DEVELOP A BETTER SPEAKING VOICE *M. Hellier*	3.00
____HOW TO MAKE A FORTUNE IN REAL ESTATE *Albert Winnikoff*	4.00
____INCREASE YOUR LEARNING POWER *Geoffrey A. Dudley*	3.00
____MAGIC OF NUMBERS *Robert Tocquet*	2.00
____PRACTICAL GUIDE TO BETTER CONCENTRATION *Melvin Powers*	3.00
____PRACTICAL GUIDE TO PUBLIC SPEAKING *Maurice Forley*	3.00
____7 DAYS TO FASTER READING *William S. Schaill*	3.00
____SONGWRITERS RHYMING DICTIONARY *Jane Shaw Whitfield*	5.00
____SPELLING MADE EASY *Lester D. Basch & Dr. Milton Finkelstein*	2.00
____STUDENT'S GUIDE TO BETTER GRADES *J. A. Rickard*	3.00
____TEST YOURSELF—Find Your Hidden Talent *Jack Shafer*	3.00
____YOUR WILL & WHAT TO DO ABOUT IT *Attorney Samuel G. Kling*	3.00

CALLIGRAPHY

____ADVANCED CALLIGRAPHY *Katherine Jeffares*	7.00
____CALLIGRAPHER'S REFERENCE BOOK *Anne Leptich & Jacque Evans*	7.00
____CALLIGRAPHY—The Art of Beautiful Writing *Katherine Jeffares*	7.00
____CALLIGRAPHY FOR FUN & PROFIT *Anne Leptich & Jacque Evans*	7.00
____CALLIGRAPHY MADE EASY *Tina Serafini*	7.00

CHESS & CHECKERS

____BEGINNER'S GUIDE TO WINNING CHESS *Fred Reinfeld*	3.00
____CHECKERS MADE EASY *Tom Wiswell*	2.00
____CHESS IN TEN EASY LESSONS *Larry Evans*	3.00
____CHESS MADE EASY *Milton L. Hanauer*	3.00
____CHESS PROBLEMS FOR BEGINNERS *edited by Fred Reinfeld*	2.00
____CHESS SECRETS REVEALED *Fred Reinfeld*	2.00
____CHESS STRATEGY—An Expert's Guide *Fred Reinfeld*	2.00
____CHESS TACTICS FOR BEGINNERS *edited by Fred Reinfeld*	3.00
____CHESS THEORY & PRACTICE *Morry & Mitchell*	2.00
____HOW TO WIN AT CHECKERS *Fred Reinfeld*	3.00
____1001 BRILLIANT WAYS TO CHECKMATE *Fred Reinfeld*	4.00
____1001 WINNING CHESS SACRIFICES & COMBINATIONS *Fred Reinfeld*	4.00
____SOVIET CHESS *Edited by R. G. Wade*	3.00

COOKERY & HERBS

____	CULPEPER'S HERBAL REMEDIES *Dr. Nicholas Culpeper*	3.00
____	FAST GOURMET COOKBOOK *Poppy Cannon*	2.50
____	GINSENG The Myth & The Truth *Joseph P. Hou*	3.00
____	HEALING POWER OF HERBS *May Bethel*	3.00
____	HEALING POWER OF NATURAL FOODS *May Bethel*	3.00
____	HERB HANDBOOK *Dawn MacLeod*	3.00
____	HERBS FOR COOKING AND HEALING *Dr. Donald Law*	2.00
____	HERBS FOR HEALTH—How to Grow & Use Them *Louise Evans Doole*	3.00
____	HOME GARDEN COOKBOOK—Delicious Natural Food Recipes *Ken Kraft*	3.00
____	MEDICAL HERBALIST *edited by Dr. J. R. Yemm*	3.00
____	NATURAL FOOD COOKBOOK *Dr. Harry C. Bond*	3.00
____	NATURE'S MEDICINES *Richard Lucas*	3.00
____	VEGETABLE GARDENING FOR BEGINNERS *Hugh Wiberg*	2.00
____	VEGETABLES FOR TODAY'S GARDENS *R. Milton Carleton*	2.00
____	VEGETARIAN COOKERY *Janet Walker*	4.00
____	VEGETARIAN COOKING MADE EASY & DELECTABLE *Veronica Vezza*	3.00
____	VEGETARIAN DELIGHTS—A Happy Cookbook for Health *K. R. Mehta*	2.00
____	VEGETARIAN GOURMET COOKBOOK *Joyce McKinnel*	3.00

GAMBLING & POKER

____	ADVANCED POKER STRATEGY & WINNING PLAY *A. D. Livingston*	3.00
____	HOW NOT TO LOSE AT POKER *Jeffrey Lloyd Castle*	3.00
____	HOW TO WIN AT DICE GAMES *Skip Frey*	3.00
____	HOW TO WIN AT POKER *Terence Reese & Anthony T. Watkins*	3.00
____	SECRETS OF WINNING POKER *George S. Coffin*	3.00
____	WINNING AT CRAPS *Dr. Lloyd T. Commins*	3.00
____	WINNING AT GIN *Chester Wander & Cy Rice*	3.00
____	WINNING AT POKER—An Expert's Guide *John Archer*	3.00
____	WINNING AT 21—An Expert's Guide *John Archer*	5.00
____	WINNING POKER SYSTEMS *Norman Zadeh*	3.00

HEALTH

____	BEE POLLEN *Lynda Lyngheim & Jack Scagnetti*	3.00
____	DR. LINDNER'S SPECIAL WEIGHT CONTROL METHOD *P. G. Lindner, M.D.*	1.50
____	HELP YOURSELF TO BETTER SIGHT *Margaret Darst Corbett*	3.00
____	HOW TO IMPROVE YOUR VISION *Dr. Robert A. Kraskin*	3.00
____	HOW YOU CAN STOP SMOKING PERMANENTLY *Ernest Caldwell*	3.00
____	MIND OVER PLATTER *Peter G. Lindner, M.D.*	3.00
____	NATURE'S WAY TO NUTRITION & VIBRANT HEALTH *Robert J. Scrutton*	3.00
____	NEW CARBOHYDRATE DIET COUNTER *Patti Lopez-Pereira*	1.50
____	QUICK & EASY EXERCISES FOR FACIAL BEAUTY *Judy Smith-deal*	2.00
____	QUICK & EASY EXERCISES FOR FIGURE BEAUTY *Judy Smith-deal*	2.00
____	REFLEXOLOGY *Dr. Maybelle Segal*	3.00
____	REFLEXOLOGY FOR GOOD HEALTH *Anna Kaye & Don C. Matchan*	3.00
____	YOU CAN LEARN TO RELAX *Dr. Samuel Gutwirth*	3.00
____	YOUR ALLERGY—What To Do About It *Allan Knight, M.D.*	3.00

HOBBIES

____	BEACHCOMBING FOR BEGINNERS *Norman Hickin*	2.00
____	BLACKSTONE'S MODERN CARD TRICKS *Harry Blackstone*	3.00
____	BLACKSTONE'S SECRETS OF MAGIC *Harry Blackstone*	3.00
____	COIN COLLECTING FOR BEGINNERS *Burton Hobson & Fred Reinfeld*	3.00
____	ENTERTAINING WITH ESP *Tony 'Doc' Shiels*	2.00
____	400 FASCINATING MAGIC TRICKS YOU CAN DO *Howard Thurston*	3.00
____	HOW I TURN JUNK INTO FUN AND PROFIT *Sari*	3.00
____	HOW TO WRITE A HIT SONG & SELL IT *Tommy Boyce*	7.00
____	JUGGLING MADE EASY *Rudolf Dittrich*	2.00
____	MAGIC FOR ALL AGES *Walter Gibson*	4.00
____	MAGIC MADE EASY *Byron Wels*	2.00
____	STAMP COLLECTING FOR BEGINNERS *Burton Hobson*	2.00

HORSE PLAYERS' WINNING GUIDES

____	BETTING HORSES TO WIN *Les Conklin*	3.00
____	ELIMINATE THE LOSERS *Bob McKnight*	3.00
____	HOW TO PICK WINNING HORSES *Bob McKnight*	3.00

____HOW TO RAISE AN EMOTIONALLY HEALTHY, HAPPY CHILD *A. Ellis*	4.00
____SEX WITHOUT GUILT *Albert Ellis, Ph.D.*	5.00
____SEXUALLY ADEQUATE MALE *Frank S. Caprio, M.D.*	3.00

MELVIN POWERS' MAIL ORDER LIBRARY

____HOW TO GET RICH IN MAIL ORDER *Melvin Powers*	10.00
____HOW TO WRITE A GOOD ADVERTISEMENT *Victor O. Schwab*	15.00
____MAIL ORDER MADE EASY *J. Frank Brumbaugh*	10.00
____U.S. MAIL ORDER SHOPPER'S GUIDE *Susan Spitzer*	10.00

METAPHYSICS & OCCULT

____BOOK OF TALISMANS, AMULETS & ZODIACAL GEMS *William Pavitt*	5.00
____CONCENTRATION—A Guide to Mental Mastery *Mouni Sadhu*	4.00
____CRITIQUES OF GOD *Edited by Peter Angeles*	7.00
____DREAMS & OMENS REVEALED *Fred Gettings*	3.00
____EXTRA-TERRESTRIAL INTELLIGENCE—The First Encounter	6.00
____FORTUNE TELLING WITH CARDS *P. Foli*	3.00
____HANDWRITING ANALYSIS MADE EASY *John Marley*	3.00
____HANDWRITING TELLS *Nadya Olyanova*	5.00
____HOW TO UNDERSTAND YOUR DREAMS *Geoffrey A. Dudley*	3.00
____ILLUSTRATED YOGA *William Zorn*	3.00
____IN DAYS OF GREAT PEACE *Mouni Sadhu*	3.00
____KING SOLOMON'S TEMPLE IN THE MASONIC TRADITION *Alex Horne*	5.00
____LSD—THE AGE OF MIND *Bernard Roseman*	2.00
____MAGICIAN—His training and work *W. E. Butler*	3.00
____MEDITATION *Mouni Sadhu*	5.00
____MODERN NUMEROLOGY *Morris C. Goodman*	3.00
____NUMEROLOGY—ITS FACTS AND SECRETS *Ariel Yvon Taylor*	3.00
____NUMEROLOGY MADE EASY *W. Mykian*	3.00
____PALMISTRY MADE EASY *Fred Gettings*	3.00
____PALMISTRY MADE PRACTICAL *Elizabeth Daniels Squire*	4.00
____PALMISTRY SECRETS REVEALED *Henry Frith*	3.00
____PROPHECY IN OUR TIME *Martin Ebon*	2.50
____PSYCHOLOGY OF HANDWRITING *Nadya Olyanova*	3.00
____SUPERSTITION—Are you superstitious? *Eric Maple*	2.00
____TAROT *Mouni Sadhu*	6.00
____TAROT OF THE BOHEMIANS *Papus*	5.00
____WAYS TO SELF-REALIZATION *Mouni Sadhu*	3.00
____WHAT YOUR HANDWRITING REVEALS *Albert E. Hughes*	2.00
____WITCHCRAFT, MAGIC & OCCULTISM—A Fascinating History *W. B. Crow*	5.00
____WITCHCRAFT—THE SIXTH SENSE *Justine Glass*	4.00
____WORLD OF PSYCHIC RESEARCH *Hereward Carrington*	2.00

SELF-HELP & INSPIRATIONAL

____DAILY POWER FOR JOYFUL LIVING *Dr. Donald Curtis*	3.00
____DYNAMIC THINKING *Melvin Powers*	2.00
____EXUBERANCE—Your Guide to Happiness & Fulfillment *Dr. Paul Kurtz*	3.00
____GREATEST POWER IN THE UNIVERSE *U. S. Andersen*	5.00
____GROW RICH WHILE YOU SLEEP *Ben Sweetland*	3.00
____GROWTH THROUGH REASON *Albert Ellis, Ph.D.*	4.00
____GUIDE TO DEVELOPING YOUR POTENTIAL *Herbert A. Otto, Ph.D.*	3.00
____GUIDE TO LIVING IN BALANCE *Frank S. Caprio, M.D.*	2.00
____HELPING YOURSELF WITH APPLIED PSYCHOLOGY *R. Henderson*	2.00
____HELPING YOURSELF WITH PSYCHIATRY *Frank S. Caprio, M.D.*	2.00
____HOW TO ATTRACT GOOD LUCK *A. H. Z. Carr*	4.00
____HOW TO CONTROL YOUR DESTINY *Norvell*	3.00
____HOW TO DEVELOP A WINNING PERSONALITY *Martin Panzer*	3.00
____HOW TO DEVELOP AN EXCEPTIONAL MEMORY *Young & Gibson*	4.00
____HOW TO OVERCOME YOUR FEARS *M. P. Leahy, M.D.*	3.00
____HOW YOU CAN HAVE CONFIDENCE AND POWER *Les Giblin*	3.00
____HUMAN PROBLEMS & HOW TO SOLVE THEM *Dr. Donald Curtis*	4.00
____I CAN *Ben Sweetland*	5.00
____I WILL *Ben Sweetland*	3.00
____LEFT-HANDED PEOPLE *Michael Barsley*	4.00
____MAGIC IN YOUR MIND *U. S. Andersen*	5.00

MAGIC OF THINKING BIG *Dr. David J. Schwartz* 3.00
MAGIC POWER OF YOUR MIND *Walter M. Germain* 4.00
MENTAL POWER THROUGH SLEEP SUGGESTION *Melvin Powers* 3.00
NEW GUIDE TO RATIONAL LIVING *Albert Ellis, Ph.D. & R. Harper, Ph.D.* 3.00
OUR TROUBLED SELVES *Dr. Allan Fromme* 3.00
PSYCHO-CYBERNETICS *Maxwell Maltz, M.D.* 3.00
SCIENCE OF MIND IN DAILY LIVING *Dr. Donald Curtis* 3.00
SECRET OF SECRETS *U. S. Andersen* 5.00
SECRET POWER OF THE PYRAMIDS *U. S. Andersen* 5.00
STUTTERING AND WHAT YOU CAN DO ABOUT IT *W. Johnson, Ph.D.* 2.50
SUCCESS-CYBERNETICS *U. S. Andersen* 4.00
10 DAYS TO A GREAT NEW LIFE *William E. Edwards* 3.00
THINK AND GROW RICH *Napoleon Hill* 3.00
THREE MAGIC WORDS *U. S. Andersen* 5.00
TREASURY OF COMFORT *edited by Rabbi Sidney Greenberg* 5.00
TREASURY OF THE ART OF LIVING *Sidney S. Greenberg* 5.00
YOU ARE NOT THE TARGET *Laura Huxley* 4.00
YOUR SUBCONSCIOUS POWER *Charles M. Simmons* 5.00
YOUR THOUGHTS CAN CHANGE YOUR LIFE *Dr. Donald Curtis* 4.00

SPORTS
BICYCLING FOR FUN AND GOOD HEALTH *Kenneth E. Luther* 2.00
BILLIARDS—Pocket • Carom • Three Cushion *Clive Cottingham, Jr.* 3.00
CAMPING-OUT 101 Ideas & Activities *Bruno Knobel* 2.00
COMPLETE GUIDE TO FISHING *Vlad Evanoff* 2.00
HOW TO IMPROVE YOUR RACQUETBALL *Lubarsky, Kaufman, & Scagnetti* 3.00
HOW TO WIN AT POCKET BILLIARDS *Edward D. Knuchell* 4.00
JOY OF WALKING *Jack Scagnetti* 3.00
LEARNING & TEACHING SOCCER SKILLS *Eric Worthington* 3.00
MOTORCYCLING FOR BEGINNERS *I. G. Edmonds* 3.00
RACQUETBALL FOR WOMEN *Toni Hudson, Jack Scagnetti & Vince Rondone* 3.00
RACQUETBALL MADE EASY *Steve Lubarsky, Rod Delson & Jack Scagnetti* 3.00
SECRET OF BOWLING STRIKES *Dawson Taylor* 3.00
SECRET OF PERFECT PUTTING *Horton Smith & Dawson Taylor* 3.00
SOCCER—The game & how to play it *Gary Rosenthal* 3.00
STARTING SOCCER *Edward F. Dolan, Jr.* 3.00
TABLE TENNIS MADE EASY *Johnny Leach* 2.00

TENNIS LOVERS' LIBRARY
BEGINNER'S GUIDE TO WINNING TENNIS *Helen Hull Jacobs* 2.00
HOW TO BEAT BETTER TENNIS PLAYERS *Loring Fiske* 4.00
HOW TO IMPROVE YOUR TENNIS—Style, Strategy & Analysis *C. Wilson* 2.00
INSIDE TENNIS—Techniques of Winning *Jim Leighton* 3.00
PLAY TENNIS WITH ROSEWALL *Ken Rosewall* 2.00
PSYCH YOURSELF TO BETTER TENNIS *Dr. Walter A. Luszki* 2.00
SUCCESSFUL TENNIS *Neale Fraser* 2.00
TENNIS FOR BEGINNERS *Dr. H. A. Murray* 2.00
TENNIS MADE EASY *Joel Brecheen* 2.00
WEEKEND TENNIS—How to have fun & win at the same time *Bill Talbert* 3.00
WINNING WITH PERCENTAGE TENNIS—Smart Strategy *Jack Lowe* 2.00

WILSHIRE PET LIBRARY
DOG OBEDIENCE TRAINING *Gust Kessopulos* 4.00
DOG TRAINING MADE EASY & FUN *John W. Kellogg* 4.00
HOW TO BRING UP YOUR PET DOG *Kurt Unkelbach* 2.00
HOW TO RAISE & TRAIN YOUR PUPPY *Jeff Griffen* 2.00
PIGEONS: HOW TO RAISE & TRAIN THEM *William H. Allen, Jr.* 2.00

*The books listed above can be obtained from your book dealer or directly from
Melvin Powers. When ordering, please remit 50¢ per book postage & handling.
Send for our free illustrated catalog of self-improvement books.*

Melvin Powers
12015 Sherman Road, No. Hollywood, California 91605

Notes

Notes

Notes

Notes